Table of Contents

Practice Test #1

Practice Questions

1. Which type of herpes virus is normally latent (does not cause disease) unless the immune system is damaged?
    a. Herpes simplex I
    b. Epstein-Barr virus
    c. Cytomegalovirus
    d. Herpes zoster

2. A dental assistant can be exposed to hazardous chemicals in the dental practice by which routes?
    a. Skin
    b. Inhalation
    c. Ingestion
    d. All of the above

3. Hepatitis has multiple bloodborne strains that may appear in healthcare settings. Which of the following is one of these strains?
    a. Hepatitis A
    b. Hepatitis E
    c. Hepatitis PV
    d. Hepatitis C

4. Which of the following is classified as a communicable disease?
    a. Xerostomia
    b. Herpes simplex type 1
    c. Influenza A
    d. Both B and C

5. _____ is the leading cause of death from infectious disease worldwide.
    a. H1N1
    b. West Nile virus
    c. Tuberculosis
    d. Malaria

6. What is the current treatment for black hairy tongue?
    a. There is no treatment for this harmless condition
    b. Frequent brushing and tongue scraping to remove excess papillae
    c. A 10-day course of antibiotics
    d. Antiseptic mouthwashes three times per day

7. Kaposi's sarcoma is a cancer that causes which of the following?
    a. Red or purple patches of abnormal skin in the mouth or throat, which contain cancer and blood cells
    b. Yellowish patches in the mouth with visible sores around the border
    c. White specks on the tongue that contain cancer cells
    d. Black spots on the soft palate and the throat

8. Oral candidiasis is caused by a fungus, which is considered:
   a. an opportunistic infection.
   b. an infestation of algae-like plaque.
   c. a spirochete.
   d. a form of hepatitis.

9. Which of the following is an appropriate armamentarium for placement of a rubber dam?
   a. Explorer, ligatures, rubber dam punch, rubber dam forceps, assorted clamps, and scissors
   b. Mirror, explorer, plastic instrument, floss, and rubber dam forceps with clamps
   c. Rubber dam punch, dams, dam forceps, wooden wedges, and clamps
   d. Mirror, rubber dam forceps, floss, gauze, and clamps

10. Dental workers are exposed to which of the following at a much higher rate than the general public?
    a. Hepatitis
    b. HIV
    c. Psoriasis
    d. *Legionella*

11. What is the best way to protect a patient from possible contaminants in dental unit water?
    a. Use high volume evacuation during procedures that require high-speed handpieces
    b. Place a rubber dam
    c. Use waterline treatments weekly
    d. Have a saliva ejector ready to evacuate all excess water during preparations

12. Antimicrobial hand sanitizer must be at least _____% alcohol to be effective in killing bacteria commonly found on the hands.
    a. 20%
    b. 30%
    c. 45%
    d. 60%

13. What is one significant difference between contact and irritant dermatitis?
    a. Irritant dermatitis is treatable with systemic antibiotics
    b. Contact dermatitis is caused by an immunologic response to latex use in the office
    c. Frequent and thorough hand washing will prevent irritant dermatitis
    d. Latex gloves are the best prevention against viral dermatitis

14. Which quadrant of the rubber dam would be chosen to punch for an endodontic treatment of tooth #21?
    a. Upper right
    b. Lower right
    c. Upper left
    d. Lower left

15. What is the primary cause of a rubber dam's failure to prevent internal contamination?
    a. Puncture of the dam by a bur or instrument
    b. Use of non-latex dams
    c. Too large of a hole punched in relation to the size of the isolated tooth
    d. The dam not being stretched tight enough

16. Where are bacteria most likely to be left behind when performing hand washing?
    a. On the back of the hands
    b. In the nail beds
    c. At the base of the thumb area
    d. None of these

17. How often should disposable plastic suction traps be changed in the dental office?
    a. Once a week
    b. Once a month
    c. Quarterly
    d. Twice each year

18. The "chain of asepsis" begins and ends with which member of the dental team?
    a. The dentist
    b. The office manager
    c. The hygienist
    d. The assistant

19. During a procedure, what item should be ready to easily prevent cross contamination when additional gauze squares are needed?
    a. A moist cotton tip applicator
    b. An explorer
    c. A sterile cotton forceps
    d. A length of floss

20. Hard surfaces within _____ from the patient chair must be disinfected.
    a. 12 inches
    b. 24 inches
    c. 3 feet
    d. 6 feet

21. Why is hand washing necessary after gloves have been removed?
    a. Latex glove use contributes to sensitivities
    b. Long-term glove use results in dermatitis
    c. No gloves are completely impermeable and can have micro-tears
    d. Perspiration naturally builds up inside gloves

22. Why is a mask put on before donning of gloves?
    a. It is more convenient to start at the top of the body and work downward when preparing for a procedure
    b. A mask can be reused if it is placed carefully
    c. Gloves may come in contact with hair and facial skin if they are put on first
    d. There is no specific reason given for this step

23. What is the proper way to proceed when a patient cannot tolerate the rubber dam placement due to anxiety issues during endodontic therapy?
    a. Use cotton isolation to protect gum tissue and the surrounding teeth
    b. Rinse the tooth frequently with chlorhexidine
    c. Apply topical anesthetic around the affected tooth
    d. Treatment cannot be completed without the use of a rubber dam

24. The use of disposable items in dentistry is an issue with regard to what global concern?
    a. The overuse of plastic packaging in the United States
    b. Non-reusable items being thrown away and ending up in landfills
    c. The chemicals and water needed to clean and sanitize staff uniforms
    d. All of these are correct

25. When working on a young patient, a(n) _____ can be used to prevent sudden closing of the jaw.
    a. mirror
    b. long cotton roll
    c. bite block/prop
    d. anesthetic

26. What items can protect patients from aerosolized spray during treatment?
    a. Safety goggles
    b. High volume evacuators
    c. Rubber dams
    d. All of these

27. Operatory keyboards are best cleaned by what method?
    a. Spraying with an all-purpose cleaner
    b. Disinfecting with wipes containing quaternary ammonia
    c. Applying soap and water with a damp towel
    d. Disinfecting with gauze saturated with alcohol

28. How does a dental assistant protect the patient from waterborne diseases during oral surgery?
    a. Spray chlorhexidine into the open socket, bone, or incision
    b. Flush the water lines before and after patient treatment
    c. Use the saliva ejector in the back of the mouth during treatment
    d. Utilize water treatment filtration

29. Digital x-ray sensors are used on multiple patients per day. How are these kept in aseptic condition?
    a. Providing continuous wipe downs with alcohol
    b. Replacing sensors 2-3 times per year to prevent bioburden
    c. Soaking the sensors in a tuberculocidal solution overnight once per week
    d. Covering the sensors with a plastic sleeve during each patient use

30. Latex or non-latex gloves are a barrier for the hands of all dental professionals. Which of the following must be considered to retain the integrity of the gloves?
    a. Washing with detergents can cause "wicking" to occur
    b. The length of a person's nails should not be considered in determining size
    c. Gloves should be kept in a cool storage place no more than two months
    d. None of these are concerns

31. Infectious waste that requires special handling, neutralization, and disposal is termed:
    a. toxic material.
    b. regulated waste.
    c. contaminated waste.
    d. ordinary garbage.

32. A(n) _____ infection is one that occurs and reoccurs in a cycle of symptoms that appear and disappear in the patient.
    a. acute
    b. opportunistic
    c. noncommunicable
    d. latent

33. Which type of waste is capable of transmitting disease?
    a. Chemical waste
    b. Infectious waste
    c. Hazardous waste
    d. Toxic waste

34. What is the best prevention for hepatitis E transmission?
    a. Thorough hand scrubbing by dental and medical personnel
    b. A vaccine that is readily available
    c. Ensuring safe drinking water
    d. Use of antibacterial spray on hard surfaces

35. Which of the following is a causative factor in dental caries?
    a. Patients whose diets include leafy, green vegetables
    b. The presence of *Streptococcus mutans* in the mouth
    c. The accumulation of blood and pus beneath the gums
    d. Patients who follow the recommended dental regimen and see their dentist every 4 to 6 months

36. Prions were discovered through the research of Dr. Stanley Prusiner who was studying Creutzfeldt-Jakob disease. What is a prion?
    a. A strain of DNA that has been damaged by radiation treatments
    b. A proteinaceous infectious particle
    c. A form of spirochete that thrives in dental water lines
    d. A particularly strong viral strain that causes flu-like symptoms

37. Oral surgery requires the use of what solution in the mouth?
   a. Surgical milk
   b. Isopropyl alcohol
   c. Sterile water
   d. Purified water

38. The Centers for Disease Control and Prevention recommend flushing of main water lines to reduce what growth?
   a. Mineral build up
   b. Waterborne viruses from patient saliva
   c. Biofilm
   d. Planktonic microbial counts

39. In the correct order, the proper steps in instrumentation sterilization are:
   a. rinsing, packaging or wrapping, and autoclaving.
   b. ultrasonic cleaning, rinsing, drying, packaging, and autoclaving.
   c. scrubbing/brushing, rinsing, packaging or wrapping, and autoclaving.
   d. holding solution tank, rinsing, and autoclaving.

40. By what method is seasonal influenza most often spread?
   a. Contact with hard surfaces where the virus has been left behind
   b. Linens that have been in contact with a person who is ill from influenza
   c. Inhalation of droplets present in the air after a person nearby has just sneezed
   d. Drinking from another person's coffee cup

41. Which type of sterilizer involves the use of a toxic gas?
   a. Glutaraldehyde
   b. Ethylene oxide
   c. Dry heat transfer
   d. Static air

42. Which level of disinfection is required for counter tops in the dental operatory?
   a. Glutaraldehyde spray
   b. Household degreaser spray
   c. Alcohol wipes
   d. Surface disinfectant with tuberculocidal capability

43. The ultrasonic cleaner loosens and removes debris on instruments by which method?
   a. Creating sound waves that form bubbles to enhance the cleaning solution
   b. Transmitting light waves through water to clean instruments
   c. Heating cleaning solutions, which softens debris on dental instruments
   d. Flushing cool water over contaminated instruments to initiate cleaning

44. How often should biologic monitoring be performed in the dental practice?
   a. At least once per week
   b. Every 3 weeks
   c. Quarterly
   d. Biannually

45. Glutaraldehyde is never to be used as surface disinfectant because:
    a. it evaporates too quickly.
    b. it is an irritant to the skin, eyes, and lungs.
    c. it is unstable and needs daily preparation.
    d. it requires two hours to fully kill microorganisms.

46. What is the initial step for instrument cleaning?
    a. Rinse instruments, scrub them with a brush, and place into a holding solution
    b. Place instruments in an ultrasonic cleaner for processing
    c. Rinse instruments and wrap them for processing in an autoclave
    d. Wrap instruments in an approved sterilization wrap

47. What is the main disadvantage to using ethylene oxide sterilization?
    a. The gas is toxic if not handled properly
    b. The process takes far too long to be efficient in a private practice
    c. The sterilization unit is too small for use in a private practice
    d. There is no disadvantage to this safe and complete sterilization method

48. When is biologic monitoring especially important and necessary?
    a. Once per month as mandated
    b. After a needle-stick injury
    c. Whenever blood or body fluids contaminate instruments
    d. For any cycle with implantable instruments

49. At what temperature does a dry heat sterilizer work best, and for how long is its typical cycle?
    a. 375 °F, 12 minutes
    b. 250°F, 30 minutes
    c. 320° F, 60-120 minutes
    d. 270° F, 20 minutes

50. All of the following are reasons for a sterilizer to fail a spore test, except when:
    a. the sterilizer becomes overloaded with cassettes and instruments.
    b. cloth wrap is in the chemical vapor sterilizer.
    c. there is a sterilizer timer malfunction.
    d. liquids (not water) were placed in a dry heat sterilizer.

51. When instruments are emerging from the ultrasonic unit with visible debris left on them, what is the likely problem?
    a. Cold water was used to fill the unit
    b. There is a clog in the filter
    c. The enzymatic solution was not mixed properly
    d. The unit is malfunctioning

52. What type of biological particulate is used in a biologic monitoring strip?
    a. Paramecia
    b. Endospores
    c. Methicillin-resistant *Staphylococcus aureus* (MRSA)
    d. Influenza B virus

53. How should cloth wrapping be fastened when used for sterilizing cassettes?
  a. Safety pins
  b. Indicator tape
  c. Stapler
  d. Any of these

54. Why is the use of cloth wrapping not recommended in an unsaturated chemical vapor sterilizer?
  a. It absorbs too much chemical vapor
  b. It degrades too quickly under the heat of sterilization
  c. It can melt and stick to surgical instruments
  d. It remains wet for hours upon removal from the sterilizer

55. All of the following are examples of mechanical instrument cleaning except:
  a. ultrasonic cleaning.
  b. the instrument washer cycle.
  c. gluteraldehyde solution.
  d. the use of long-handled brushes.

56. Which type of hard surface disinfectant is broad spectrum, intermediate level, and must be prepared daily?
  a. Glutaraldehyde
  b. Synthetic phenol compounds
  c. Iodophors
  d. Chlorine dioxide

57. What CDC level of disinfectant should be used to clean surfaces not contaminated with blood?
  a. High level
  b. Intermediate level, with antimicrobial properties
  c. Intermediate level, with no tuberculocidal activity
  d. Low level

58. Unsaturated chemical vapor, used in some sterilizers, consists of what components?
  a. Isopropyl alcohol and ethylene glycol
  b. Sodium sulfate and denatured water
  c. Water and isopropyl alcohol
  d. Formaldehyde and alcohol

59. In order to assure patients that instrumentation is sterilized, it is important:
  a. to open instrument packs and do a thorough hand washing after the patient is seated.
  b. to use a new pair of gloves when recording patient notes.
  c. to change amalgam separator filtration once or twice per year.
  d. to display licenses and certification near patient operatories.

60. Surgical instruments require _____ to insure they are not corroded by thorough and constant sterilization under high heat and pressure.
  a. soaking for at least an hour in detergent
  b. placement in a surgical milk bath before packaging for the autoclave
  c. thorough scrubbing with brushes
  d. extra rinsing with hot water

61. Which of the following instruments should never be stored unwrapped in a drawer?
    a. Slow-speed handpiece
    b. Hemostat
    c. Bone file
    d. Syringe

62. Radiographic film packets can be disinfected by which method?
    a. Dipping them in water before processing
    b. Wiping carefully with a sanitizing wipe
    c. Placing them in a glutaraldehyde solution for one minute
    d. No disinfection is needed once the outside sleeve is removed

63. How are sink handles kept free of debris and contaminants when needed during patient treatment?
    a. Continuous wiping with disinfectants
    b. Barrier tape
    c. Plastic bag covering
    d. Any of these are acceptable

64. Why is it important to have heavy-duty utility gloves in the sterilization area?
    a. Water used to rinse instruments is quite hot and could cause burns
    b. To protect healthcare workers' hands from puncture injuries during cleaning
    c. In case an inspection team needs to see where they are kept
    d. They are used for window washing and floor cleaning

65. Which of these statements is true about surface covers in the dental operatory?
    a. They can be reused if the item was untouched during the procedure.
    b. They are too costly to be used to cover all potentially exposed items.
    c. All surfaces that cannot be repeatedly pre-cleaned and disinfected must have barriers.
    d. None of these are true

66. One important step in the chain of asepsis that is often overlooked is which of the following?
    a. Using a new mask for each day
    b. Autoclaving of cassettes
    c. Storage of chemicals in a cool, dark space
    d. Pre-cleaning to reduce bioburden

67. When pre-cleaning of hard surfaces is performed, what technique is best for removing bioburden?
    a. Wipe with disinfectant wipes, allow it to dry, and then repeat
    b. Spray with disinfectant and wipe with paper towels
    c. Wipe with a paper towel and spray if still visibly soiled
    d. Clean with alcohol wipes, then allow to air dry

68. When changing the filtration on vacuum suctions, remember the following:
    a. Filters can be soaked in bleach overnight and reused
    b. Personal protective equipment is required
    c. If daily suction cleaning solution is used, it should be changed every three months
    d. One-size filters can be trimmed to fit any vacuum line

69. Aseptic technique can be maintained while making notations in patient charts. How is this accomplished?
    a. Spraying paper charts with antiseptic mist
    b. Using barrier protection on writing implements
    c. Changing gloves after writing notes
    d. None of these are true

70. Surface disinfection can be done by an iodophor-type cleaner. Which category is this?
    a. Sterilant
    b. High level
    c. Intermediate level
    d. Low level

71. OSHA's law that pertains to an employee's "Right-To-Know" is officially called the:
    a. Hazard Communication Standard.
    b. SDS for Employees.
    c. Employee Rights in the Workplace.
    d. Hazardous Material Identification for Employees.

72. A Hazard Communication Standard must contain which of the following?
    a. Employee training, a written program, and SDS for every chemical in the practice
    b. Labeling information for chemicals in the practice, a written program, and a manual for recordkeeping
    c. A written program and manual for recordkeeping and government regulation information
    d. OSHA safety labels

73. When a chemical spill has occurred in the dental office, it is important to remember to:
    a. use protective eyewear and utility gloves and to keep neutralizing agents on hand.
    b. notify all staff and keep a record of the incident.
    c. dispose of all hazardous materials immediately.
    d. All of these are correct

74. During an oral surgery, a dental assistant is sprayed in the face with aerosolized water and blood. What is the next step for this assistant?
    a. The assistant should wipe her gloves and goggles before returning to the procedure
    b. The assistant must leave the operatory for the rest of the procedure
    c. The dentist will have to file an exposure report for this incident
    d. The assistant must step out of the procedure, remove her gloves, mask, and eyewear, and replace it with new PPE (personal protective equipment) before returning to the chairside.

75. What is the proper response to a patient who is having difficulty breathing in the dental chair?
    a. Give the patient a tablet of nitroglycerin sublingually and monitor his blood pressure
    b. Activate the medical emergency plan: call 911 emergency services and begin CPR if necessary
    c. Give oxygen through a mask and scavenger system
    d. Take the patient's pulse and blood pressure

76. After giving an anesthetic to the patient, she begins to sweat and says that her heart is beating fast. You notice that she has red blotches on her arms. What type of medical situation is likely to be occurring?
    a. Seizure
    b. Cardiac arrest
    c. An allergic reaction
    d. Insulin secretion response

77. Which of the following statements is true about disposable dental items?
    a. It is acceptable to reuse high volume suctions if they are disinfected between patients.
    b. Whenever patient items cannot be sterilized, they should be in single-use, disposable form.
    c. Disposable saliva ejectors are completely safe as long as patients close their lips tightly and draw fluid in.
    d. Non-sterile gauze can be used in a surgical procedure.

78. What type of information can be found on a Safety Data Sheet?
    a. Information on the physical or chemical characteristics of a material used in a dental practice
    b. Fire and explosion hazard data
    c. Boiling point of a given chemical or material
    d. All of these are correct

79. An instrument that penetrates bone or soft tissue is classified by the CDC as:
    a. noncritical.
    b. semicritical.
    c. critical.
    d. hazardous.

80. The fire extinguishers in a dental practice are in compliance if maintained by what method?
    a. The expiration date must be within the past two years
    b. They are checked and professionally serviced annually
    c. Any fire extinguishers must bear the official seal of OSHA
    d. Extinguishers should be mounted near an exit

81. In order to practice safe handling, dental workers must be sure to do which of the following?
    a. Use sharps containers as intended and not allow them to be overfilled
    b. Use sturdy brushes to clean up broken glass
    c. Place radiographic films in a covered garbage receptacle as soon as the patient has left the practice
    d. None of these are correct

82. What is the rationale for keeping two separate refrigerators in the dental practice?
    a. Convenience for staff members and patients
    b. Separation of dental materials and chemicals from food and drink
    c. More storage space for dental chemicals used in the office
    d. Cost efficiency rather than off-site storage of chemicals

83. What type of information is useful for healthcare workers in limiting exposure to potentially hazardous chemicals?
    a. The flammability of hazardous chemicals
    b. The expiration date of hazardous chemicals
    c. The smell, appearance, and labeling information of chemicals used in the office
    d. The chemical composition of hazardous chemical mixes

84. _____ must be provided for staff and patients, including having fume hoods in laboratory spaces.
    a. Masks and shoe covers
    b. Adequate ventilation
    c. Fresh water
    d. Utility gloves

85. OSHA has a system for determining inspection priority for dealing with any situation. What are the components of this system?
    a. Imminent danger, catastrophe/ fatal accident, complaints, and programmed inspection
    b. Fatality, complaints, and referrals from reported incidents
    c. Imminent danger, accident with or without chemical exposure, and safety violations
    d. Each situation is evaluated on its own to determine corrective action

86. How does an office demonstrate that they have complied with the necessary recordkeeping in the event of a needle-stick injury to a staff member?
    a. A log of phone calls to emergency medical personnel is required
    b. Produce copies of the employee's immunization records and infection control/safety training certificates
    c. Show the inspector the location and date of exposure and record of said incident
    d. None of these

87. In what year was OSHA created to regulate and enforce workplace safety laws?
    a. 1971
    b. 1978
    c. 1982
    d. 1984

88. How many employees in a dental office will necessitate a written emergency action plan?
    a. 2 or more
    b. 5 or more
    c. 11 or more
    d. 20 or more

89. All of the following are the employer's responsibility according to OSHA except:
    a. tornado and hurricane protection spaces.
    b. fire extinguisher maintenance.
    c. laundering of employee uniforms off site.
    d. medical emergency kits.

90. By what method is a written infection control program evaluated?
   a. OSHA-required annual training
   b. Appropriate equipment is being used
   c. The office assesses the infection control methods used by healthcare staff
   d. All of the above

91. What is the required amount of time a dental practice must retain an employee's medical record regarding immunization and post-exposure medical evaluation?
   a. 5 years
   b. 10 years
   c. 7 years past the termination of employment
   d. 30 years past the termination of employment

92. _____ is a necessary record to be maintained in the dental practice.
   a. Disposal of hazardous waste
   b. Storage of topical anesthetic
   c. Laboratory asepsis
   d. Instrument processing

93. A specific area of the dental practice must be set aside for:
   a. the cleaning and sterilization of instruments.
   b. employees to change from street clothing to uniform attire.
   c. a patient restroom.
   d. storage of lab jackets.

94. Each dental practice must have a(n) _____ designated to maintain and keep the written hazard communication standard.
   a. area
   b. staff member
   c. document
   d. desk

95. Which type of documentation is required for a chemical that is mixed in the office by a healthcare worker?
   a. Written notice of past inspections
   b. A list of known chemical hazards in the office
   c. Safety Data Sheets from the manufacturer
   d. Digital copy of the chemical make up on a CD-ROM for review

96. Under the OSHA statutes, _____ must be informed and trained in safe handling of chemicals.
   a. all persons over 18 years old
   b. administrative staff
   c. patients
   d. new and contract employees

97. Labeling of potentially hazardous chemicals includes a diamond symbol showing which of the following?
- a. Yellow, blue, and green sections to facilitate recognition
- b. Health hazards, flammability, and reactivity of the chemical
- c. Health hazards and chemical mixing ratios for office use
- d. None of these are correct

98. In order to comply with OSHA's Laboratory standard, a(n) _____ is a necessary element.
- a. oxygen tank
- b. disposable brush head
- c. chemical hygiene plan
- d. sharps container

99. When is it necessary to activate the emergency action plan, written in the Hazard Communication Standard?
- a. Once per month, for training purposes
- b. After the practice has opened for the first time
- c. When a medical emergency has occurred
- d. In the event of a fire at the dental office

100. What is one of the most important elements of any infection control program?
- a. Regular review by the dentist to ensure timely updates and training
- b. Maintenance of the written plan in a clean binder near the patient charts
- c. Purchasing of all written materials directly from the OSHA website
- d. Daily mixing of disinfectant cleaners in the laboratory

Answers and Explanations

1. **C: Cytomegalovirus.** The virus is normally latent, but may become active in a person who is immunocompromised. Once active, it is highly contagious and transmitted through most bodily fluids. Care of the immunocompromised patient must be a serious consideration in any healthcare setting, since his body's systems are already damaged and susceptible to opportunistic infections.

2. **D: All of the above.** Dental assistants must be aware of chemicals entering the body through the skin, through breathing aerosols or drinking from contaminated water sources, or through eating food that may also be contaminated. This is important to maintaining personal health and for the safety of the community.

3. **D: Hepatitis C.** There are five types of hepatitis that have been discovered and extensively studied. Three of these (B, C, and D) are chronic infections. A good way to remember which ones are transmitted through fecal-oral routes is that those strains are represented by vowels (A and E), whereas the strains represented by consonants (B, C, and D) are transmitted percutaneously and through the mucosal tissues. These strains are also known as bloodborne strains of hepatitis.

4. **D: Both B and C.** Influenza A (swine flu) and herpes simplex I are both communicable diseases; they are spread from person to person and are not genetic or congenital diseases. Xerostomia is a condition of lacking saliva in the mouth. It is commonly seen in patients who have undergone radiation therapy or those who take a large amount of daily medications.

5. **C: Tuberculosis.** This disease is a considerable threat to healthcare workers, those with HIV-positive status, and any patient with a weakened immune system. The rod-shaped bacterium of tuberculosis can withstand many disinfectants that kill less tenacious germs. For this reason, a disinfectant's time to kill bacteria is measured by how fast it can eliminate tuberculosis on any surface.

6. **A: There is no treatment for this harmless condition.** According to the Mayo Clinic, black hairy tongue is a harmless condition that requires no treatment. It is generally caused by a dramatic change in the bacterial counts inside the mouth. This can be related to such factors as recent antibiotic use, poor oral hygiene, breathing through the mouth; using medications containing bismuth (such as Pepto Bismol), regular use of mouthwashes containing oxidizing agents (such as peroxide) or astringent agents (such as witch hazel), and heavy tobacco use.

7. **A: Red or purple patches of abnormal skin in the mouth or throat, which contain cancer and blood cells.** The other answers are descriptions referencing symptoms of other conditions. Kaposi's sarcoma is most often seen in patients who are HIV-positive or those who have AIDS.

8. **A: An opportunistic infection.** *Candida albicans,* the fungus responsible for candidiasis, is known to infect those whose immune systems are already damaged or their suppression capabilities have been eroded by age or disease. It is common among those with HIV, and is treated with prescription anti-fungal oral lozenges or anti-fungal pills such as Diflucan (fluconazole).

9. **A: Explorer, ligatures, rubber dam punch, rubber dam forceps, assorted clamps, and scissors.** The floss, gauze, wedges, and plastic instruments listed in the other available choices may or may not be useful in placement of a rubber dam on the patient. The scissors are used to adjust the dam by

- 19 -

removing the area of latex that sits around or near the nose (for enhanced patient breathing and comfort) and for quick removal of the dam after treatment is complete.

10. D: *Legionella*. These bacteria are encountered by dental health care workers on a daily basis due to exposure to aerosolized spray during procedures. *Legionella* is not usually a major concern for dental workers, unless they or their patients are immunocompromised.

11. B: Place a rubber dam. The best way to protect the patient from contaminants in dental unit water is to place a rubber dam at the beginning of the procedure. High volume evacuator (HVE) use is helpful, but it is best to keep all aerosols and water droplets from touching the patient's mouth and skin.

12. D: 60%. In order to be effective, antimicrobial hand sanitizer must be at least 60% alcohol. This is a fact that is put forth by the Centers for Disease Control and Prevention. Most hand sanitizers formulated for healthcare workers include moisturizers to prevent drying of the skin and subsequent itching from dermatitis.

13. B: Contact dermatitis is caused by an immunologic response to latex use in the office. This allergic reaction can range from an itchy rash to severe anaphylaxis. Irritant dermatitis is caused by frequent hand washing and failure to thoroughly rinse and dry the skin after washing.

14. B: Lower right. Before punching a rubber or non-latex dam, it is important to estimate the position of the tooth to be treated when the dam is in place. The use of a rubber stamp with the following shape: can help train new dental staff to locate the proper quadrant before using the

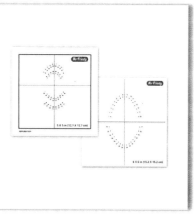

punch.

15. C: Too large of a hole punched in relation to the size of the isolated tooth. It is best to use the smallest hole punch that the tooth size and clamp will allow. Too large of a hole may cause gapping or tearing around the coronal part of the tooth. Moisture can then contaminate the dry field. Whether or not the dam is stretched tightly, the field should remain dry. Non-latex dams are just as safe to use against internal contamination as the natural latex rubber type. It is rare that an instrument will puncture the dam, but occasionally the bur may nick or cut the material.

16. B: In the nail beds. The most common area that bacteria can still be found after hand washing is under and around the nail beds. This area can harbor dangerous bacteria that can grow especially potent under acrylic nails. It is for this reason that healthcare workers are not allowed to wear acrylic nails, nor any nail lacquer of any kind.

17. B: Once a month. Changing disposable suction traps once a month is a minimum amount of time since the traps tend to fill up with the removal of many amalgam fillings or old crowns. If this is not done regularly, the suction hoses can back up and their waste materials start to come out, even when turned on.

18. D: The assistant. The dental assistant is charged with a very important duty to begin the chain of asepsis each day, and like a circle, to continue to maintain it each and every day. It is this devotion to duty that makes the dental assistant's position such an important part of the healthcare community.

19. C: A sterile cotton forceps. A cotton tip is never completely clean if it has water on it, and an explorer is not likely to hold onto gauze when removing it from its covered container. Dental offices should keep several cotton forceps ready for this purpose. Floss would not be useful in this case.

20. C: 3 feet. Every item within three feet is subject to being sprayed with aerosolized bacteria during patient treatment. This is a very specific distance that should guide every decision about whether to disinfect a surface or piece of equipment or to cover it with a plastic barrier. It is necessary to use a surface disinfectant that contains tuberculocidal additives on any counter tops within three feet of the dental chair. These surfaces are near enough to the patient's mouth to be contaminated by aerosol back spray.

21. C: No gloves are completely impermeable and can have micro-tears. All gloves have some level of breathability to them to be comfortable for dental assistants to wear for long procedures. This means that microscopic bacteria from blood and saliva can enter and potentially expose the wearer to bloodborne pathogens.

22. C: Gloves may come in contact with hair and facial skin if they are put on first. There is a reason why gloves and masks are put on in a specific order. Hair and skin both contain oils, which can be transferred to the gloves before patient treatment if the mask is put on secondarily. Masks can never be reused on another patient once they have been in a procedure.

23. D: Treatment cannot be completed without the use of a rubber dam. Endodontic specialists and general dentists everywhere are never supposed to initiate or complete endodontic therapy unless the patient is protected by rubber dam isolation. If the patient cannot tolerate the feeling of this safety device, then anti-anxiety measures such as nitrous oxide or oral medications may be necessary. The patient always has the choice to opt out of treatment entirely.

24. D: All of these are correct. Attempts to make dentistry more "green" are always associated with global concerns. The answers listed are all considerations, and only the future will tell what compromises can be made. The use of disposables is a blessing of convenience and safety for healthcare in general, but it does have an environmental cost.

25. C: Bite block/prop. These safety devices are designed to prevent the patient from sudden movement or closure during the dental procedure. They are typically used as a resting point for the jaw muscles, but in a very young patient, they become a safety device to avoid cutting the tongue or tissue during handpiece use. An anesthetic would probably not be useful in this case because it would cause the patient to have even more difficulty judging whether the jaw is open or closed.

26. D: All of these. Safety goggles, high volume evacuators, and rubber dams are all ways to protect the patient from aerosolized spray, which can contain bloodborne pathogens that transmit disease.

27. B: Disinfecting with wipes containing quaternary ammonia. The use of technological items in the dental operatory creates an infection control issue. The quaternary ammonia wipes typically have a tuberculocidal quality that makes them a good choice for cleaning keyboards and digital sensors, if permitted by the manufacturer. Alcohol is never recommended because it dries out the plastic keys and casings, causing cracks to occur. Avoid spraying any type of cleaner on the keys since the water content can damage the key function.

28. B: Flush the water lines before and after patient treatment. Flushing the lines is the best defense against waterborne diseases that grow in the dark, moist environment of the dental tubing. Use of the saliva ejector during oral surgery procedures is never recommended because of the back pressure that can be created when the patient closes his lips around it. Water treatment filters are a great way to keep water clean at the source, but they cannot do anything to combat what is already growing in the tubing connected to the patient chair.

29. D: Covering the sensors with a plastic sleeve during each patient use. Sensors should never be wiped with alcohol since this can cause cracking in the cords and damage to the sensor itself. They should never be soaked in any type of solution for disinfection. These digital components are very costly to replace and most practices must train every staff member to handle them with care.

30. A: Washing with detergents can cause "wicking" to occur. There are inherent defects in the natural material of gloves that can be exploited by opportunistic bacteria seeking a host. A dental staff member must be careful not to let her nails grow too long or wear any kind of jewelry that may puncture or cause micro-tears in the gloves.

31. B: Regulated waste. Regulated waste must be handled with specific care to assure it is neutralized and disposed of in the safest possible way. This protects the dental office staff, patients, and the community as a whole. The differences between these types of waste are as follows:

Types of waste

Waste and by-products cover a diverse range of materials, as the following list illustrates (percentages are approximate values):

 Infectious waste: waste contaminated with blood and its by-products, cultures and stocks of infectious agents, waste from patients in isolation wards, discarded diagnostic samples containing blood and body fluids, infected animals from laboratories, and contaminated materials (swabs, bandages) and equipment (disposable medical devices).
 Sharps: syringes, needles, disposable scalpels and blades, etc.
 Chemicals: solutions such as mercury, solvents, and disinfectants.
 Pharmaceuticals: expired, unused, and contaminated drugs, vaccines and sera.
 Radioactive waste: items such as glassware contaminated with radioactive diagnostic material or radiotherapeutic materials.
 Heavy metals waste: items such as broken mercury thermometers.

(World Health Organization, 2011)

---

32. D: Latent. This type of infection will have acute symptoms that manifest themselves, then disappear and reappear again. Examples of latent infections are cold sores and genital herpes.

33. B: Infectious waste. Hazardous waste poses a risk to humans, but is not necessarily infectious (i.e. broken glass). Toxic waste is defined as that which is poisonous, so it is deadly, and not a transmitter of disease. Please refer to the info-graphic in the answer to number 31.

34. C: Ensuring safe drinking water. Hepatitis E is not a chronic condition, but it is spread through the fecal-oral transmission route. There is no vaccine for this type of hepatitis. This means that safe drinking water and well-regulated and maintained sanitation is necessary for its reduction within the community. Antibacterial sprays are not the first line of defense against this type of infection.

35. B: The presence of *Streptococcus mutans* in the mouth. *Streptococcus mutans* forms a capsule that allows it to survive the body's attempts to eradicate it. This makes it particularly virulent and capable of causing serious disease. As an example, this bacterium can be passed from mother to child by kissing or sharing eating utensils with an infant whose teeth are still developing.

36. B: A proteinaceous infectious particle. Prions are composed entirely of proteins that lack nucleic acids (DNA or RNA). It was discovered that proteins alone can transmit diseases like spongiform encephalopathy (mad cow disease). A prion is not a spirochete and is highly resistant to heat, chemical agents, and irradiation. There is no treatment for the diseases caused by prions, so the best prevention is not to eat contaminated foods, especially those that contain nerve tissue.

37. C: Sterile water. This type of water is always required for use in the mouth during any oral surgery procedure. Purified water may not be sterilized, but may be cleaner than regular city water. Isopropyl alcohol cannot be used directly in the mouth due to the sensitivity of oral mucosa. Surgical milk is a rust-proofing solution used to coat surgical instruments before sterilization in an autoclave.

38. D: Planktonic microbial counts. The Centers for Disease Control and Prevention recommend flushing dental water lines to diminish the levels of planktonic microbial bacteria found in water. However, flushing the dental lines should not be the sole method of improving water quality in the dental office.

39. B: Ultrasonic cleaning, rinsing, drying, packaging, and autoclaving. The steps of sterilization must be consistently followed in order to assure that instruments are sterile, and to facilitate the consistent training of newly hired dental assistants and office staff.

40. C: Inhalation of droplets present in the air after a person nearby has just sneezed. Droplets that hang in the air after an infected person has sneezed or coughed are the most common route of transmission of influenza (also called flu). The best way to prevent infection is to be vaccinated every year just before the start of the flu season, and to remember to thoroughly wash hands and surfaces regularly in the home, at work, and at school.

41. B: Ethylene oxide. This type of sterilizer involves the use of toxic gases. It is not commonly found in private practices due to the 16 hours of aeration required after sterilization is complete. The units needed to perform ethylene oxide sterilization are very large and frequently used in hospitals or very large clinics. The correct answer must be a concern for the staff and patients of the dental practice. The toxic gas used in this type of sterilization is a danger to dental office staff and is very rare in private practices.

42. D: Surface disinfectant with tuberculocidal capability. It is necessary to use a surface disinfectant that contains tuberculocidal additives on any counter tops within three feet of the dental chair. These surfaces are near enough to the patient's mouth to be contaminated by aerosol back spray.

43. A: Creating sound waves that form bubbles to enhance the cleaning solution. The ultrasonic cleaner creates sound waves, which cause bubbles to implode. This mechanical action compliments the chemical action of the cleaning solution.

44. A: At least once per week. This type of monitoring is essential to prove that a sterilization system is performing properly. Some types are read in the office, while others can be sent out for testing in an offsite location. There are several other reasons for biological monitoring: after an electrical or power outage, after changing packaging materials (to verify that items are sterilized), after training new employees, and once a week to verify proper functioning of the autoclave. It is perfectly acceptable to use biological monitoring more often than once per week to check that patient items are sterile.

45. B: It is an irritant to the skin, eyes, and lungs. Glutaraldehyde is never used as a surface disinfectant because it is a skin, eye, and lung irritant. Its evaporation time has no bearing on its use as a surface disinfectant, since it takes a minimum of six hours to be effective, depending on its concentration.

46. B: Place instruments in an ultrasonic cleaner for processing. This initial step in sterilization processing can include the use of a holding solution to prevent blood from drying on instruments. Hand scrubbing with a brush or sponge is never ideal because of the risk of puncture injuries to dental staff. Instruments cannot be wrapped for the autoclave until they have had debris removed, washed, and rinsed off.

47. A: The gas is toxic if not handled properly. The toxic gas used in ethylene oxide sterilization is a danger to dental office staff, and is very rare in private practices. The large clinics and hospitals that use ethylene oxide sterilization have to allow a minimum of 16 hours of post-processing time to aerate the instruments. While answer B might be true in this case, the larger concern must be for the dental office staff and patients.

48. D: For any cycle with implantable instruments. There are several other reasons for biological monitoring: after an electrical or power outage, after changing packaging materials to verify that items are sterilized, after training new employees, and once a week to verify proper functioning of the autoclave. It is perfectly acceptable to use biological monitoring more often than once per week to check that patient items are sterile.

49. C: 320°F, 60-120 minutes. This chart shows the difference in temperature and time needed for all types of sterilizers.

Type of Sterilization	Standard Sterilizing Conditions
Steam Autoclave	250°F for 20-30 minutes
Unsaturated Chemical Vapor	270°F for 20 minutes
Dry Heat Oven	320°F for 60-120 minutes
Rapid Heat Transfer	375°F for 12 minutes

50. D: Liquids (not water) were placed in a dry heat sterilizer. All of the answers are correct reasons for sterilization failure except for the last one. Liquids cannot be placed in the chemical vapor because sterilizing agents cannot penetrate solutions and in the dry heat sterilizer, solutions will boil over and evaporate (Miller, 2010).

51. D: The unit is malfunctioning. Ultrasonic units clean the gross debris from instruments through the use of sound waves, which create bubbles in the water. The bubbles burst and the implosions result in a percussive effect on the soiled instruments. Holding a piece of aluminium foil in the water for 20 seconds will show if the bubbles are capable of removing debris as desired. The temperature of the water is not important, and the enzymatic solution should not cloud the water.

52. B: Endospores. The bacteria found in biological monitoring strips are a harmless strain of heat-resistant spores. These are the toughest organisms to kill; therefore, they are a great test of an autoclave's sterilization capabilities.

53. B: Indicator tape. This type of tape is specifically designed to withstand the heat of the sterilization process and contains a color-changing medium that allows for verification of the cycle. It is never acceptable to use metal staples, paper clips, or safety pins in the wrapping of instruments due to the concern for sharp objects that could potentially penetrate the packaging or cloth material.

54. A: It absorbs too much chemical vapor. Cloth wrapping absorbs so much vapor in the unsaturated chemical sterilizer that it becomes a hazard to dental office staff. It is much preferred that the paper or plastic peel pouches are used for this purpose. The use of unsaturated chemical vapor means that no water will remain on the wrappings, so answer D is not of concern in this case.

55. C: Glutaraldehyde solution. Mechanical cleaning of contaminated instruments implies the use of some type of contact with the surface that scrubs it clean. A holding solution or gluteraldehyde ("cold sterile") solution works without contacting the surface in an abrasive or penetrating fashion. Long-handled brushes are the only acceptable type for hand scrubbing instrumentation, but this is the least desirable method due to the risk of injury from punctures.

56. B: Synthetic phenol compounds. These types of surface disinfectants are prepared daily and are classified as intermediate-level hospital disinfectants. Since they leave a chemical residue on some surfaces, it is best to use synthetic phenol compounds on rubber or plastic items, rather than metals.

57. D: Low level. Low-level disinfectants are used for surfaces that have not been contaminated with blood. The ideal types of disinfectants will have residual activity that continues long after evaporation leaves the surface dry. It is necessary to use a surface disinfectant that contains tuberculocidal additives on any counter tops within three feet of the dental chair.

58. D: Formaldehyde and alcohol. These components make up the unsaturated chemical vapors used in this type of sterilization. Unsaturated chemical vapors are used in place of water to sterilize instruments and the instruments then dry quickly following processing.

59. A: To open instrument packs and do a thorough hand washing after the patient is seated. Patient surveys often return with comments pertaining to the value of actually seeing the instrument pack opened in front of them and watching the healthcare workers perform thorough hand washings. All

jewelry should be removed and the nails should be cleaned as part of this process. A patient's sense of comfort and peace of mind is enhanced when he feels that the staff truly cares for his best health outcomes.

60. B: Placement in a surgical milk bath before packaging for the autoclave. Detergents may remove some of the surface sheen on surgical tools and contribute to the oxidizing formation of rust. It is acceptable to use regular dish washing soap as a holding solution for oral surgery instruments, but they should be dipped in surgical milk (without subsequent rinsing) to coat them before packaging for the autoclave. This will protect their longevity.

61. C: Bone file. Since this instrument's purpose is to file down rough, exposed bone surface during an oral surgery procedure, it is considered a critical instrument. This classification means that it must be treated with the utmost care and autoclaved on the longest cycle. Care should also be taken to make sure unused surgical instruments are resterilized every two months to be sure the packaging material has not been compromised, allowing dust and aerosols inside.

62. B: Wiping carefully with sanitizing wipe. Any kind of submersion of film packets, such as in water or glutaraldehyde solution, could compromise the emulsifying layer on the film itself. Removing the outside sleeve in the operatory would mean destroying the latent image on the film, so this is not an option for disinfecting film packets.

63. D: Any of these are acceptable. Reduction of bioburden, which is a microscopic build-up of patient blood and saliva on hard surfaces that are often difficult to clean, is always a concern in order to prevent cross contamination in the dental operatory. This is a universal practice for all dental offices.

64. B: To protect healthcare workers' hands from puncture injuries during cleaning. This is an OSHA safety regulation that must be practiced in all dental offices. It does not matter if an inspector is there to check or not. All contaminated instruments should be treated as potentially hazardous while in the sterilization area. Typically, heavy-duty utility gloves are not used for cleaning floors and windows; standard rubber household gloves are acceptable for these chores.

65. C: All surfaces that cannot be repeatedly pre-cleaned and disinfected must have barriers. This is a standard practice for all dental offices. Reduction of bioburden (a microscopic build-up of patient blood and saliva on hard surfaces that are often difficult to clean) is always a concern in order to prevent cross contamination in the dental operatory.

66. D: Pre-cleaning to reduce bioburden. Using a new mask each day, autoclaving of cassettes, and storing chemicals in a cool, dark place may all be common practices for a dental assistant, but pre-cleaning of areas that can accumulate bioburden are often overlooked in the course of a busy day.

67. A: Wipe with disinfectant wipes, allow it to dry, and then repeat. The steps of operatory sanitation and disinfection must be consistently followed in order to assure that instruments are sterile and to facilitate the training of new office staff.

68. B: Personal protective equipment is required. The filters on vacuum system tubing are highly contaminated with bacteria and dental assistants must wear their personal protective equipment (PPE). Filters should be placed in a biohazard-labeled container and disposed of according to the state guidelines established for hazardous and regulated waste. The filters cannot be reused and every dental unit manufacturer has a specific size designed for use on their units.

69. B: Using barrier protection on writing implements. All surfaces that cannot be repeatedly pre-cleaned and disinfected must have barriers. Barrier protection can be used on writing utensils as a method of maintaining aseptic technique.

70. C: intermediate level. Iodophor-type cleaners cannot be used for sterilization, but are useful as surface disinfectants. Pre-cleaning of units is recommended to reduce the levels of bioburden in the operatory. This step is often overlooked in the interest of saving time, but it is very important for office infection control practices.

71. A: Hazard Communication Standard. The Hazard Communication Standard is the official name for OSHA's law that provides an employee's "Right To Know." This law provides the identification of chemicals and the hazards associated with acute exposures in the workplace. The Employee Rights in the Workplace details information relating to wages, work schedules, and the rights that are retained upon termination.

72. A: Employee training, a written program, and SDS for every chemical in the practice. OSHA's Hazard Communication Standard actually contains five parts in its entirety: a written program, inventory of hazardous chemicals, SDS for every chemical, proper labelling of containers, and employee training. One member of the staff must be designated as the person responsible for this program.

73. D: All of these are correct. All of the listed answers are important to know and to have in a written plan in case of spills in the dental office. The hazardous spill should always be cleaned immediately, and care should be taken not to allow the incident to happen again. There is no limit to the number of reports that can be submitted, but it is the duty of all healthcare personnel to use standard precautions to prevent accidental spills.

74. D: The assistant must step out of the procedure, remove her gloves, mask, and eyewear, and replace it with new PPE (personal protective equipment) before returning to the chairside. It is not acceptable to just wipe down goggles and gloves after being sprayed with aerosolized water and blood. It is not necessary to file an exposure report unless there has been a needle-stick injury or an accident resulting from a hazardous condition in the office itself.

75. B: Activate the medical emergency plan: call 911 emergency services and begin CPR if necessary. A patient's breathing difficulties can be an early sign of a much more serious situation. The heart could develop an abnormal rhythm, such as tachycardia or other cardiac arrhythmia. It is always safer to activate emergency medical services (EMS) and allow emergency professionals to address and handle this type of incident.

76. C: An allergic reaction. Although a reaction to anesthesia is rare, common reactions will manifest as hives, nausea, and dizziness. Injectable epinephrine should be available in the office medical emergency kit to be administered subcutaneously in this situation. Diphenhydramine, which may reverse some of the effects of an allergic reaction, is also available in pill form.

77. B: Whenever patient items cannot be sterilized, they should be in single-use, disposable form. Attempts to make dentistry more "green" are consistently facing this type of question. The answers listed are all considerations, and only the future will tell what compromises can be made. The use of disposables is a blessing of convenience and safety for healthcare in general, but it does have an environmental cost.

78. D: All of these are correct. Health hazards, flammability, and reactivity of the chemical, as well as its boiling point, are all contained within the Safety Data Sheets. The hazardous ingredients and the health hazard data of the chemical or material are also listed on an SDS.

79. C: Critical. This type of instrument requires sterilization due to its very high risk of disease transmission. Examples of critical items include scalpels, bone chisels, and burs. Commonly used plastic items, which cannot be sterilized, should be purchased in disposable form to facilitate disease prevention in the office. This classification means that items must be treated with the utmost care and autoclaved on the longest cycle.

80. B: They are checked and professionally serviced annually. For safety, the fire extinguishers should be visible and easily accessible to the office staff. Certain staff members should also be trained in how to operate them to put out small office fires. This person's name should be listed in a written office emergency plan. It is not necessary to mount them near an exit.

81. A: Use sharps containers as intended and not allow them to be overfilled. Sharps containers should be "point of use," which means they are as close as possible to the area where sharps are being removed and ready to be discarded. Tongs, rather than sturdy brushes, are the proper implements to clean up pieces of broken glass. This minimizes the risk of a sharps injury in the office.

82. B: Separation of dental materials and chemicals from food and drink. Certain materials such as composites, sealant material, and bonding agents will require refrigeration to maximize their potency and longevity. Office staff should have another place to store their food and drink without risk of contamination by chemical agents.

83. C: The smell, appearance, and labeling information of chemicals used in the office. Knowing the smell and appearance of a potential chemical spill could help office staff to identify when an accidental leak has occurred. It will also confirm what type of safety measures to enact or which authorities to contact.

84. B: Adequate ventilation. This is very important for office safety and staff comfort when it comes to the mixing of chemicals and lab materials. Materials such as rubber base for impressions or acrylic for custom trays and temporary restorations can cause sufficient odors to fill the office. These fumes may also trigger headaches and breathing issues for those with respiratory difficulties such as asthma.

85. A: Imminent danger, catastrophe/fatal accident, complaints, and programmed inspection. This protocol has been established to allow for a systematic method of prioritizing the thousands of reports OSHA receives each year. There are many follow-up steps for offices that receive an inspection visit. The documentation must be clear and fair to eliminate bias and to represent the spirit of the laws that OSHA is enforcing.

86. B: Produce copies of the employee's immunization records and infection control/safety training certificates. The rationale behind this is so that if a person contracts a disease as a result of the needle-stick injury, legal records will be available to verify that the former staff member was vaccinated or treated at the time of exposure. If he had already been treated for the disease or condition during his tenure at the office, this can be a legal defense point for the office or the victim's claims in any future legal action.

87. A: 1971. The Occupational Safety and Health Administration (OSHA) was created by a mandate from President Richard Nixon, who signed it into law on December 29, 1970. OSHA's mission is to "assure safe and healthful working conditions for working men and women by setting and enforcing standards and by providing training, outreach, education and assistance." OSHA has developed a number of training, compliance assistance, and health and safety recognition programs throughout its history. The OSHA Training Institute, which trains government and private sector health and safety personnel, began in 1972. OSHA started the Voluntary Protection Programs in 1982, which allow employers to apply as "model workplaces" to achieve special designation if they meet certain requirements.

88. C: 11 or more. According to OSHA, a written plan must be kept in office records if the office employs 11 or more people. This is the size where OSHA mandates have decreed the need for certain documentation, which must be enacted and maintained.

89. C: Laundering of employee uniforms off site. OSHA does not have specific laws in place concerning where employee uniforms are laundered. Employees should arrive with enough time to change into clean scrubs before the start of each shift. If a laundry service is available, the uniform scrubs can be taken off site in closed biohazard bags for cleaning and disinfection if they have been exposed to blood or body fluids.

90. D: All of the above. OSHA-required annual training, use of appropriate equipment, and the office's assessment of the infection control methods used by healthcare staff on a regular basis are all parts of evaluating an effective infection control program. Any good protocol needs to be reviewed periodically to see where improvements can be made and updates added. Annual office training should be conducted to review the general practices and provisions.

91. D: 30 years past the termination of employment. The rationale behind this is so that if a person contracts a disease later found to be caused by the chemicals found in a particular dental office, legal records can be located to see if the former staff member was vaccinated or treated at the time of exposure.

92. A: Disposal of hazardous waste. The disposal of hazardous waste record is one of the required documents to be contained in the OSHA files of the dental office. Records of all chemicals stored in the practice should also be filed with this document to show the chain of responsibility.

93. A: The cleaning and sterilization of instruments. It is safest for all concerned if a designated area is reserved for the cleaning and sterilization of contaminated instruments. This area must not be in a common hallway. It should be well ventilated but contain no windows, which can create a problem with dust if left open.

94. B: Staff member. One staff member must be designated in the Hazard Communication Standard to be responsible for keeping the written program organized and up to date. This person is also named as the contact point in the office when updates become digitally available online or in print versions.

95. C: Safety Data Sheets from the manufacturer. A Safety Data Sheet (SDS) is a document that contains information on the potential hazards (health, fire, reactivity, and environmental), as well as how to work safely with the chemical product. It is intended to provide workers and emergency

personnel with procedures for handling or working with that substance in a safe manner, and includes information such as physical data (melting point, boiling point, flash point, etc.), toxicity, health effects, first aid, reactivity, storage, disposal, protective equipment, and spill-handling procedures (Wikipedia, 2013).

96. D: New and contract employees. The SDS must be readily available to the health and safety committee or representative, as well as to the workers who could be exposed to the controlled product. If a controlled product is made in the workplace, the employer has a duty to prepare an SDS. Employers may computerize the SDS information as long as all employees have access. Employees must also be trained on how to use the computer, the computers must be kept in working order, and the employer must make a hard copy of the SDS available to the employee or the safety and health committee upon request. (Occupational Health and Safety Administration, 2013)

97. B: Health hazards, flammability, and reactivity of the chemical. Chemical mixing ratios are not contained on the safety stickers and signage; that information can be found in the manufacturer's pamphlets. OSHA designed the stickers to allow for quick assessments of chemicals and to know if a risk exists if two chemicals are stored in close proximity to each other.

98. C: Chemical hygiene plan. OSHA's Hazard Communication Standard contains five parts in its entirety: A written program, inventory of hazardous chemicals, SDS for every chemical, proper labeling of containers, and employee training. One member of the staff must be designated as the person responsible for this program.

99. D: In the event of a fire at the dental office. There is no practical need to activate the emergency plan when opening a new practice. The Hazard Communication Standard specifies that the plan should contain the following: procedures for reporting fire or other emergency, evacuation procedures, accounting for all employees after evacuation is completed, rescue and medical duties for personnel who are to perform them, names and contact information for those who can be contacted for further information.

100. A: Regular review by the dentist to ensure timely updates and training. Any good protocol needs to be reviewed periodically to see where improvements can be made and updates added. Annual office training should be conducted to go over the general practices and provisions, as well as to add new items.

Practice Test #2

Practice Questions

1. During which stage of an infectious disease is the infected individual most contagious to dental healthcare workers?
    a. Convalescent stage
    b. Acute stage
    c. Prodromal stage
    d. Incubation stage

2. Which of the following terms can be defined as a person who is infected with a disease but does not show any recognizable symptoms of that disease?
    a. Pathogenic carrier
    b. Microbial carrier
    c. Communicable carrier
    d. Asymptomatic carrier

3. Which concept states that all human blood and body fluids, including excretions and secretions, are to be treated as if they are infected with a bloodborne disease?
    a. Standard precautions
    b. Universal precautions protocol
    c. Prodromal prevention concept
    d. Blood-borne pathogen standard

4. Which of the following infections may occur when dental healthcare workers are exposed to infected dental unit waterlines and aerosolized water?
    a. Tetanus
    b. Legionnaires' disease
    c. Methicillin-resistant *Staphylococcus aureus* (MRSA)
    d. Hepatitis B

5. When working on a patient who is infected with syphilis, the dental assistant must ensure that she is adequately protected by personal protective equipment in order to prevent which of the following that is associated with this infection?
    a. An infectious ulcerating sore called a chancre
    b. Inhalation of highly infectious viral particles known as *Treponema pallidum*
    c. Exposure to bacteria that will lead to an infection causing lockjaw
    d. An infectious lesion on the tongue called herpes

6. Which of the following is a severe allergic reaction that may be experienced by the patient or the dental healthcare worker in response to the latex proteins that are found in latex gloves?
    a. Latex Allergy type 1
    b. Latex Allergy type 2
    c. Latex Allergy type 3
    d. Latex Allergy type 4

7. What is the main reason as to why occupational infections with hepatitis B among dental healthcare workers have decreased in the past 30 years?
   a. An increase in the number of dentists and other dental healthcare workers becoming vaccinated
   b. A decrease in the number of patients that are infected with infectious diseases
   c. Enhancements in the design of dental sterilization units
   d. Implementation of the OSHA Hazard Communications Standard

8. If a patient is infected with a communicable disease when receiving dental treatment, which of the following is recommended for use to aid in the prevention of that infection?
   a. Cotton roll holders
   b. Dry angles
   c. The small suction
   d. The high volume evacuator

9. Which is an example of a chronic condition that affects the liver and is spread by blood transfusions and organ transplants?
   a. Shingles
   b. Herpes type 1
   c. Hepatitis A
   d. Hepatitis C

10. Which of the following is a correct statement regarding the hepatitis B vaccine?
   a. If a dental healthcare worker declines the vaccination, he or she must sign a declination waver form.
   b. The vaccine is not effective after 5 years and the CDC recommends a booster dose after that time.
   c. When given, the vaccine introduces the body to hepatitis B antibodies, which lead the body to forming hepatitis B antigens.
   d. The vaccination is given as a series of 2 injections, spaced out over a period of 8 months.

11. Which of the following statements is incorrect regarding hand washing and gloving in the dental office?
   a. Hands should be dry prior to donning gloves to prevent the growth of bacteria underneath the gloves.
   b. It is preferred that treatment rooms have "hands-free" sinks to avoid cross-contamination.
   c. The dental healthcare worker may use liquid soap or bar soap to wash hands prior to a general restorative procedure.
   d. Hands must be washed after removing gloves due to small unapparent defects that may be present.

12. Which of the following statements best describes the use of alcohol-based hand rubs in dentistry?
   a. They are waterless antiseptic agents that are more effective than plain soap at reducing the microbial flora found on the hands.
   b. They are agents that are new to the market and are made to be used in place of antimicrobial hand scrubs prior to surgical procedures.
   c. Alcohol concentrations in alcohol-based hand scrubs work most effectively with 40-50% alcohol.
   d. These products are indicated for use when the dental healthcare worker's hands are visibly soiled or contaminated with biological matter.

13. What type of products are not intended for use with latex gloves due to their ability to break down the latex and compromise the effectiveness of the product?
   a. Antimicrobial surgical scrubs
   b. Alcohol-based hand rubs
   c. Petroleum-based products
   d. Non-dental scented lotion products

14. According to the CDC, which of the following is a correct general recommendation for proper hand hygiene in the field of dentistry?
   a. Keep natural nail tips shorter than ½ inch.
   b. Do not wear artificial nails, as they may harbor an increased number of bacteria.
   c. Do not use hand lotions or creams after washing hands, as this may decrease the integrity of the gloves.
   d. The dental healthcare worker should wash his hands for a minimum of one minute prior to a general restorative procedure.

15. Which of the following is correct regarding the use of masks in the dental office?
   a. Wearing a standard dental mask will protect the dental healthcare worker against 90% of microbes that come into contact with that mask.
   b. The dental healthcare worker should change his mask with every patient.
   c. When processing dental instruments, the dental healthcare worker does not need to wear a mask.
   d. It is common for dental offices to use N-95 respirators when patients come in with upper respiratory infections.

16. When considering the use of protective eyewear when working chairside, which of the following is correct?
   a. The dental healthcare worker may substitute a face shield in place of eyewear when working chairside.
   b. Eyewear is an optional piece of protective equipment that must be provided by the employer.
   c. It is recommended that protective eyewear be sanitized thoroughly only at the end of every day.
   d. It is uncommon for the dental healthcare worker to offer eye protection to the patient and this should be avoided.

17. Which of the following is the correct order for the placement of personal protective equipment?
    a. Mask, protective clothing, eyewear, gloves
    b. Eyewear, protective clothing, mask, gloves
    c. Protective clothing, eyewear, mask, gloves
    d. Mask, eyewear, protective clothing, gloves

18. When should the dental healthcare worker wear utility gloves?
    a. When exposing radiographs
    b. During laboratory procedures
    c. When processing dental instruments
    d. When performing chairside procedures

19. Which of the following are found on the hands, are permanent residents of the skin, and can't be removed with any type of hand washing or scrubbing regimen?
    a. Subcutaneous skin flora
    b. Permanent skin flora
    c. Resident skin flora
    d. Transient skin flora

20. How does the use of a dental dam help to protect the dental healthcare worker against the spread of infection?
    a. It improves access by helping to retract the lips and the tongue.
    b. It decreases the amount of aerosols emitted by the patient into the air.
    c. The dental dam protects the oral cavity from exposure to harmful microbes when there are open surgical sites.
    d. It helps to prevent the accidental swallowing of debris and excess fluids.

21. Which of the following best applies to the use of single-use or disposable devices?
    a. Certain types may be reprocessed and used on a second patient only
    b. They always come in a heat-tolerant alternative form
    c. They should only be used when a heat stable form is not available
    d. They serve as a good substitute for items that are difficult to clean

22. Which of the following is a correct statement regarding pre-procedural mouth rinses?
    a. Pre-procedural rinses are to be used both before and after the procedure for maximum effectiveness.
    b. There is a large amount of scientific evidence that supports the use and effectiveness of pre-procedural mouth rinses in preventing oral infections in patients.
    c. Pre-procedural mouth rinses are recommended by the CDC prior to prophylaxis procedures.
    d. The intent of pre-procedural mouth rinses is to reduce the amount of microbes found in the oral cavity and prevent them from being released into the air during a procedure.

23. When considering protection from laser or electrosurgery plumes or surgical smoke, which of the following is correct?

    a. Tissue debris, viruses, and odors are released into the air during the use of a laser on a patient.

    b. If viruses are found in surgical smoke, the risk of disease transmission from breathing the smoke is 80%.

    c. The dental healthcare worker is required to wear an N-95 respirator during all surgical laser or electrosurgical procedures.

    d. The CDC recommends that all dental healthcare workers exposed to smoke from electrosurgical procedures from 1998-2005 obtain HIV testing due to the high number of HIV particles found in the surgical smoke.

24. Which of the following is incorrect regarding single-dose vials of anesthetic solution used in dentistry?

    a. If there are left over contents, they should be discarded and never combined with other left over materials for reuse.

    b. They pose a risk for contamination if they are punctured repeatedly.

    c. They should be used whenever possible for parenteral medications.

    d. Medication from a single-dose syringe may be reused only of the needle on the syringe is changed.

25. When handling biopsy specimens, what should the dental healthcare worker do to decrease the chance of cross-contamination?

    a. Label the container with a hazard sticker during storage

    b. Transfer the specimen in a sturdy container with a secure lid

    c. Keep the specimen stored in the refrigerator until it is ready to ship

    d. Return the container to circulation for future specimens after the lab has performed the required testing and returned the container and results.

26. How should the dental healthcare worker handle a contaminated impression before it is sent out to the dental laboratory?

    a. It must be sterilized in a chemiclave prior to packaging.

    b. Impressions should be rinsed with warm water and soap, as intermediate-level disinfectants lead to distortion of the impression.

    c. It should be cleaned to remove any bioburden present, disinfected, rinsed, and packaged.

    d. The impression should be soaked in a high-level disinfectant for a minimum of 10 minutes and rinsed prior to packaging.

27. Which of the following is classified as a touch surface and needs to be disinfected with an intermediate-level disinfectant?

    a. Drawer handle

    b. Instrument tray

    c. Handpiece holder

    d. Countertop

28. Which of the following best describes the advantage of using a surface barrier in the dental office?
    a. Surface barriers do not add plastic waste to the environment, as many of them can be reused when disinfected properly.
    b. Surface barriers protect surfaces that are not easily cleaned and disinfected.
    c. Surface barriers have antimicrobial properties and may work to disinfect while they are in place during procedures.
    d. Surface barriers are much cheaper to use compared to the chemicals needed for pre-cleaning and disinfecting.

29. Which of the following guidelines for the use of exam gloves must be followed by the dental healthcare worker when working chairside?
    a. If the dental assistant needs to leave the treatment room during a procedure, he can continue to wear his exam gloves as long as he does not touch anything and comes back to the treatment room in a timely manner.
    b. If a glove tears during a procedure, the dental healthcare worker should wait for the best time to stop the procedure and alert the doctor that his glove is torn and needs to be changed.
    c. Change gloves frequently, once every hour, even during the same patient procedure, as the glove's integrity may become compromised from the chemicals and other items that the dental assistant is touching.
    d. The dental assistant is allowed to wash his exam gloves only if he briefly touched a contaminated object, but is still performing a non-invasive procedure on a different patient.

30. When considering the disinfection of housekeeping surfaces in the dental office, which of the following is correct?
    a. The dental assistant must ensure that walls and drapes are included in the disinfection process as well as the floors and countertops.
    b. If blood or body fluids are present, the dental assistant must use a high-level disinfectant to decontaminate the area.
    c. An EPA-registered hospital disinfectant or low-level disinfectant is recommended to clean these surfaces.
    d. Mops and cloths can be used for 3 days before they need to be cleaned and allowed to dry for reuse.

31. Which of the following is an example of regulated biohazardous waste?
    a. A used Band-Aid
    b. A piece of 2x2 gauze that has dried blood flaking off of it
    c. Used fixer solution
    d. A used patient napkin with a small amount of blood

32. Which of the following containers is the appropriate container to place extracted teeth and blood-soaked items?
    a. A labeled sharps container
    b. A hazardous waste container
    c. A biohazardous non-sharp medical waste container
    d. Any container that has the required hazardous waste symbol.

33. Which of the following should the dental healthcare worker avoid when handling sharps items in the dental office?
    a. If the sharps container is nearing full capacity, continue to fill it only until sharps items are even with the top brim of the container.
    b. Be sure to keep sharps containers at the point of use, in each operatory, and in the sterilization center.
    c. Ensure that sharps items are placed in a puncture resistant container labeled with a biohazard label.
    d. Never break or bend sharps prior to placing them into the sharps container.

34. What should the dental healthcare worker do if the outside of a biohazardous waste container becomes contaminated when items were placed inside?
    a. Use an intermediate-level disinfectant to decontaminate the outside of the biohazard bag.
    b. Remove the contents from the first bag and place into a new biohazard bag.
    c. Place the entire contaminated bag into a second biohazard bag and seal both bags.
    d. Personal protective equipment should always be used when handling biohazard bags, so no additional steps are required if this were to occur.

35. Which of the following is the appropriate container for used burs and orthodontic bands?
    a. Regular trash
    b. Biohazardous waste container
    c. Non-regulated hazardous waste container
    d. Sharps container

36. When storing dental instruments, the dental healthcare worker must avoid which of the following?
    a. Using paper and autoclave tape to wrap cassettes, as this does not keep the instruments sterile as well as the paper/plastic pouches
    b. Storing instruments in closed or covered cabinets
    c. Using a black permanent marker to record the date on the package of instruments as this will cause the marker to bleed through and stain the instruments during sterilization
    d. Placing the sterile packs on shelves under the sink in the sterilization area

37. When disposing of used fixer solution, which of the following statements is correct?
    a. Used fixer solution can be disposed of down a regular city drain, as it is safe to enter the public sewage system.
    b. Used fixer must be placed into a puncture resistant biohazardous waste container for disposal.
    c. Used fixer solution is a type of hazardous waste and must be disposed of by a commercial company who is contracted with the dental office.
    d. The dental staff must run used fixer through a filtering system at the end of every month and then the used fixer is okay to dispose of down a regular city drain.

38. Which of the following provides the best description of disease transmission by indirect contact?
    a. Performing a procedure where blood accidently splashes into the eyes of the dental healthcare worker
    b. Using a contaminated object that was not sterilized properly on a new patient
    c. Breathing in aerosols suspended in the air, which are attached to infectious microbes
    d. Being exposed to spray or spatter containing infectious microorganisms

39. Which of the following is an example of a parenteral transmission?
    a. When a person comes into contact with microbes on an inanimate surface and then transfers them to his own body.
    b. When a dental healthcare worker is exposed to a patient's blood through aerosols from the high-speed handpiece.
    c. When a patient sneezes and blood from an extraction site lands in the dental healthcare workers eye.
    d. When a dental healthcare worker accidently pokes himself with a contaminated needle.

40. How is the *Mycobacterium tuberculosis* organism spread in the dental healthcare setting?
    a. By a percutaneous exposure to infected blood
    b. When a patient or dental healthcare worker does not wash their hands after using the restroom
    c. By breathing in infectious bacteria that are present in the air
    d. By a droplet of water and blood that lands on the dental healthcare workers exposed mucosa

41. Which of the following can be described as items that touch mucous membranes in the oral cavity and need to be processed by heat sterilization and receive a high level disinfection?
    a. Critical level instruments
    b. Semi-critical instruments
    c. Midlevel critical instruments
    d. Noncritical instruments

42. Which of the following terms can be described as the destruction of all living microbes?
    a. Pre-cleaning
    b. Disinfection
    c. Decontamination
    d. Sterilization

43. Which level of disinfectants is capable of sterilization?
    a. Maximum-level
    b. High-level
    c. Intermediate-level
    d. Low-level

44. When a disinfectant claims to have a tuberculocidal time of 3 minutes, what does this mean?
    a. The disinfectant can remove most of the tuberculosis bacterium in under 3 minutes.
    b. The disinfectant can remove all of the tuberculosis bacterium and any weaker forms in 3 minutes.
    c. The disinfectant is capable of removing more resistant forms of microbes than tuberculosis in any time over 3 minutes.
    d. The disinfectant has the capability to weaken any tuberculosis bacterium present on a surface in any time over 3 minutes, making the bacterium non-infectious.

45. How should a noncritical item that is contaminated with blood be handled?
    a. The item should be placed in the ultrasonic machine for a minimum of 10 minutes.
    b. The item should be placed in a biohazardous waste container for proper disposal.
    c. The blood should be removed from the item and the item should be placed in a heat sterilizer.
    d. The item should be cleaned and disinfected with an intermediate-level disinfectant prior to its next use.

46. Which of the following is a semi-critical instrument?
    a. Scalpel
    b. Bone chisel
    c. Extraction forceps
    d. Dental handpiece

47. Which of the following is the correct processing protocol for dental handpieces?
    a. Pre-cleaned in the ultrasonic and then placed in the chemical vapor sterilization machine
    b. Soaked in a high-level disinfectant for a minimum of 10 hours
    c. Placed in the ultrasonic, wiped off with disinfectant and gauze, and placed in an ethylene oxide sterilization unit
    d. Wiped off with a disinfectant and gauze and then bagged and placed in a heat sterilization machine

48. Which of the following is an example of a noncritical instrument?
    a. Stethoscope
    b. Dental mouth mirror
    c. Impression trays
    d. Amalgam condenser

49. What is the main purpose of the holding solution?
    a. The holding solution serves as an intermediate-level disinfectant required prior to processing
    b. It provides a method of pre-cleaning prior to instrument sterilization
    c. To prevent debris from hardening onto the surface of the dental instrument
    d. It is used as a disinfectant for the dental instruments

50. Which of the following methods of sterilization uses low temperatures to sterilize items and requires 4-12 hours for sterilization and up to 16 hours for post-sterilization aeration?
    a. Stem under pressure
    b. Dry heat
    c. Unsaturated chemical vapor
    d. Ethylene oxide

51. Which of the following is the most desirable method for pre-cleaning instruments due to its effectiveness?
    a. Hand scrubbing
    b. Instrument washers
    c. Holding solution
    d. Ultrasonic machine

52. What is the best way to check the effectiveness of the ultrasonic machine?
    a. A testing strip
    b. A foil test
    c. A biological indicator
    d. Ultrasonic machine tape

53. Under what circumstances should the dental healthcare worker use the flash cycle available on most sterilization machines?
    a. When the items to be sterilized are heat-sensitive
    b. As a backup if the dental office runs out of paper/plastic pouches or instrument wrapping paper
    c. When the items in the cycle are intended for immediate use
    d. This cycle is to be used as a method of pre-cleaning dental instruments prior to being run through the regular sterilization cycle.

54. Which of the following methods of sterilization monitoring can best ensure the dental healthcare team that the sterilization machine is working properly?
    a. Biological monitoring
    b. Chemical monitoring
    c. Physical monitoring
    d. Test-strip monitoring

55. What is a second name given to biological indicators?
    a. Microbe monitoring devices
    b. Physical indicator strips
    c. Autoclave tapes
    d. Spore tests

56. Which of the following terms is best defined as the colonization of bacteria, fungi, and protozoa that live inside a protective slime layer?
    a. Biofilms
    b. Biological colonies
    c. Microbial counts
    d. *Legionella* layers

57. Which of the following CFU/mL levels is the maximum amount allowed in dentistry set by the Environmental Protection Agency?
    a. Less than 300 CFU/mL
    b. Less than 400 CFU/mL
    c. Less than 500 CFU/mL
    d. Less than 600 CFU/mL

58. Which of the following protocols must be followed to aid in the maintenance of the dental unit water lines?
    a. They should have a bleach/water mix run through them at the beginning and end of each day.
    b. They should be run for 20-30 seconds after each patient.
    c. They should be removed from the unit once per week and run through the autoclave.
    d. They should be flushed for 5 minutes at the beginning of every day.

59. Which of the following techniques should be utilized during surgical procedures in dentistry?
    a. The solutions being used must be decontaminated with an antibacterial tablet prior to use.
    b. The dental auxiliary must use distilled water when assisting in surgical procedures.
    c. The office must use a filtering system to remove bacteria and microbes in the solutions used during surgery.
    d. The office must use a sterile water delivery system or device to deliver solutions during surgery.

60. What is the correct protocol to follow if the dental office is located in a community that is under a public health department issued boil-water advisory?

    a. The dental office should avoid using water from the public water supply for all patient procedures.

    b. The dental office should boil all water used for a minimum of 30 seconds at a full boil before use.

    c. The office should not use tap water for dental procedures but it is allowed for hand washing.

    d. The dental auxiliary must not use water for invasive dental procedures, but it is allowed for routine procedures and exams.

61. What needs to be done in order to prevent cross-contamination between a dental office and a dental laboratory?

    a. Disinfect all impressions with an intermediate-level disinfectant prior to sending them to the laboratory.

    b. If metal impression trays have been used, ensure that these items have been disinfected and wiped down prior to use on the next patient.

    c. Assume the laboratory is responsible for the final disinfection of patient items and that these items have been disinfected prior to placing the items in the patient's mouth.

    d. Ensure impressions and orthodontic appliances do not come into contact with water prior to sending them to the laboratory, as this may distort the detail in these items.

62. Which of the following disinfectants are the best choices to use on alginate impressions?

    a. Complex phenols and chlorine dioxide

    b. Quaternary ammoniums and glutaraldehyde

    c. Iodophors and diluted sodium hypochlorite

    d. Phenols and iodophors

63. What is the correct protocol to follow when performing oral surgical procedures to prevent cross-contamination?

    a. The dentist must use a formulated surgical scrub prior to all invasive procedures.

    b. The dentist must use an antimicrobial soap and water rinse prior to all surgical procedures.

    c. The use of antimicrobial soap alone and rinsing with tap water is an acceptable practice.

    d. If sterile gloves are used, the dentist may use plain soap and water to wash prior to surgery.

64. What is the correct protocol to follow when considering decontamination procedures for digital x-ray sensors?

    a. After use, the sensor should be immersed in a high-level disinfectant for the time specified by the manufacturer for sterilization.

    b. The sensor should be covered during use with a barrier and then removed from the cable cord and placed in the autoclave for sterilization.

    c. The sensors should be covered with barriers during use and then disinfected with an intermediate-level disinfectant.

    d. The sensors should be placed in the autoclave sterilizer on the flash cycle after being wiped down with an intermediate-level disinfectant.

65. How should film-positioning devices used in dental radiology be decontaminated?
    a. If they are heat-tolerant, they should be sterilized using heat.
    b. Because they are critical level instruments, they need to be sterilized using a high-level disinfectant with an increased contact time specified by the manufacturer.
    c. They need to be cleaned, placed in the ultrasonic, and then placed in an immersion bath of an iodophor solution.
    d. If they are heat sensitive, the item should be sterilized only by a chemiclave, as this uses low temperatures and will not distort the item.

66. Which of the following is the most effective technique to use when attempting to reduce the chance of cross-contamination when using film-based radiographic techniques?
    a. Submerge all exposed films for 1 minute in a high-level disinfectant prior to processing.
    b. Place the film packets in the patient's mouth and then after exposure, wipe each film packet off prior to placing them into the processors.
    c. Use barriers over each film when placed in the patient's mouth and remove the barriers and film packets prior to placing the films into the processor.
    d. Remove the films from their packets and wipe down each actual film prior to placing them into the processor.

67. When decontaminating an area on the floor in a treatment room after a blood spill, which of the following should be used?
    a. A low-level disinfectant
    b. Detergent and water
    c. A hospital disinfectant that has a HBV and HIV claim
    d. An intermediate-level disinfectant that has a tuberculocidal claim

68. Which of the following is a requirement for all surface disinfectants used in dentistry?
    a. Surface disinfectants must be able to sterilize when items are submerged in them for extended periods of time.
    b. Surface disinfectants must have an HIV kill time of less than 6 minutes.
    c. Surface disinfectants must be listed on the American Dental Association's website.
    d. Surface disinfectants must have an Environmental Protection Agency registration number.

69. Which of the following is the main reason for sterilization failure in the dental office?
    a. Machine malfunction
    b. Operator error
    c. Inadequate electrical support for the machine from the outlet
    d. Insufficient cleaning and maintenance of the sterilization machine

70. Which steps must be completed once a boil-water advisory has been cancelled or lifted?
    a. Use an intermediate-level disinfectant to soak the dental unit tubing for 10 minutes.
    b. Unless otherwise directed by public officials, flush dental unit water lines for 1-5 minutes prior to use for patient care.
    c. Remove all dental hoses from the unit and place in the autoclave machine for sterilization.
    d. After public officials have lifted the advisory, the dental office can return to using tap water with no additional actions.

71. Which of the following terms best describes physical devices or items that should be used by the dental auxiliary to prevent occupational exposures to bloodborne pathogens and aid dental auxiliaries in providing safe dental care while at work?
   a. Engineering controls
   b. Work practice controls
   c. Hazardous waste controls
   d. Contamination controls

72. Who is covered by the OSHA bloodborne pathogens standard?
   a. All employees who are occupationally exposed to blood or other potentially infectious materials
   b. Anyone in any type of job, as it is a multifaceted standard
   c. Physicians and dentists are covered and have the option to delegate duties of this standard to their employees
   d. Clinical dental workers only

73. Which of the following is a correct statement regarding the exposure control plan that is part of the bloodborne pathogens standard?
   a. This is an optional safety net that many dental offices have in place to keep their workers safe.
   b. This is a document designed to eliminate or minimize employee exposure to blood or other potentially infectious materials.
   c. This is a document that is filed with OSHA by each individual dental office after it has been developed and must be approved prior to implementation.
   d. This is a document that is developed by the dentist, based on their history of patient experiences in their dental offices and is kept in a private location, separate from accessible office documents.

74. How often does the exposure control plan need to be reviewed and updated by the dental team members?
   a. Weekly
   b. Monthly
   c. Annually
   d. Only when procedures change or when new procedures are introduced

75. Which of the following provides the best description regarding what the OSHA exposure determination is?
   a. A list of all employees who have received percutaneous injuries in the past year at a specific dental clinic.
   b. An employer's requirement of identifying workers with the potential of occupational exposure to blood.
   c. A statement by each employee on what they are doing to keep themselves free of occupational exposures while at work.
   d. A dental auxiliary's way of indicating which procedures hold the highest risk of disease transmission and occupational exposures.

76. According to the bloodborne pathogens standard, which of the following is an unnecessary or unacceptable practice in the dental office?
    a. Employers need to ensure that their workers are washing their hands immediately after coming into contact with blood.
    b. Engineering controls need to be examined and maintained on a regular basis by the workers who use them.
    c. Engineering controls are required to be used to eliminate employee exposure.
    d. Employers have the option of providing hand washing stations as long as there are alcohol-based hand rubs available for workers.

77. Which is correct regarding the hepatitis B vaccination?
    a. If an employee refuses the vaccination, they are required to obtain counseling regarding the benefits of the vaccination.
    b. The employee is responsible for the cost of the vaccination if they initially decline, but change their mind in the future.
    c. If an employee starts the series but does not finish it, they are not required to because of the immunity that has been built up in their body from the initial doses of the vaccine.
    d. The employer must offer the vaccination to all employees at no cost within 10 days of initial employment.

78. When is the optimal time to receive a titer test to determine the presence of antibodies due to receiving the hepatitis B vaccine?
    a. 1 week after the 2nd dose to determine the need for the 3rd dose
    b. 1-2 months after the final dose
    c. 6 months after the series has been completed
    d. Annually

79. Which of the following is the correct action to take if an employee has received the hepatitis B vaccination series twice but has yet to demonstrate antibody production from a hepatitis B titer test?
    a. The employee should engage in a 3rd series of the hepatitis B vaccination and have a titer test 1-2 months after that has been completed.
    b. The employee should be counseled regarding precautions to prevent hepatitis B infection and the proper protocol to follow in the event of an exposure.
    c. The employee should be removed from direct patient care and placed in a position with a decreased chance of a percutaneous injury occurring.
    d. The employee should receive an alternative form of the vaccine to determine if their body will respond.

80. According to the bloodborne pathogens standard, which of the following is a correct requirement of the employer and/or employee?
    a. The employer must replace personal protective equipment used by the employees as needed at no cost to the employees.
    b. If an employee damages utility gloves due to incorrect cleaning procedures, they are required to replace the gloves in a reasonable time.
    c. The employee is responsible for laundering their personal uniforms.
    d. The employee must provide their own gloves if they are experiencing dermatitis reactions due to the gloves currently provided by the employer.

81. What is the proper protocol that should be followed in the event that there is broken glass that may be contaminated with blood or other potentially infectious materials in a dental operatory?

a. The dental auxiliary should use a brush and dustpan or tongs to pick up the items and place them into a sharps container.

b. The treatment area should be taken out of use and the items should be carefully picked up and placed into a trash receptacle that is closest to the area to eliminate the chance of a percutaneous injury to a staff member.

c. The incident exposure kit should be brought into the treatment area and the glass should be placed into the testing bags and sent to the laboratory to determine the presence of an infectious disease in order to properly counsel the staff members involved.

d. There is nothing out of the normal routine that needs to be done in this situation, the glass should be picked up and placed in a non-regulated trash bin.

82. Which of the following is an example of infectious waste that may be found in the dental office setting?

a. A patient napkin that has a small amount of blood on it from a restorative procedure.

b. A 2x2 gauze that has dried blood that is flaking off of the gauze.

c. A Band-Aid that was worn and removed by a patient during patient care.

d. A cotton roll that was used to increase visibility in the oral cavity during an extraction.

83. Which is NOT included in the bloodborne pathogens standard protocol that should be followed when cleaning contaminated work surfaces at the dental office?

a. Contaminated work surfaces should be decontaminated with an appropriate disinfectant after completion of a procedure.

b. A contaminated area should be cleaned at the end of the work shift if the surface has been contaminated since the last cleaning was completed.

c. An area should be cleaned immediately following a spill of blood or any other potentially infectious material.

d. If there is saliva spatter on a work surface contaminating the surface, the procedure should be halted and the area should be cleaned.

84. Which of the following types of dental waste should be placed in containers that are closable, and constructed to contain all contents and prevent leakage of fluids during handling, storage, transport, and shipping?

a. General waste

b. Contaminated waste

c. Infectious waste

d. Specialized waste

85. When handling contaminated laundry, which of the following protocols needs to be followed by the dental staff member?

a. Employees who handle the contaminated laundry should wear protective gloves and other appropriate personal protective equipment when necessary.

b. If there is wet laundry, this should avoid contact with any type of bag due to the potential of soak-through and should be placed immediately into the washing machine.

c. All laundry generated by a dental office must be shipped to an off-site secondary facility in order to prevent cross-contamination.

d. The dentist is the only staff member that is able to process or handle contaminated laundry due to the liabilities that can occur if there was an occupational exposure from items found in the laundry area.

86. Following a report of an exposure incident at the dental office, what does the employer need to do for the exposed employee?

a. The employer should allow the employee 5 days of paid vacation to seek the medical care that the employee deems necessary.

b. The employer must document the incident and provide the affected employee with a confidential verbal and written warning and place this in the employee's permanent work history.

c. The employer is responsible for alerting all staff members at the office in order to prevent cross-contamination from the potentially infected employee.

d. The employer should provide the employee with a confidential medical evaluation and follow up by a qualified physician.

87. According to the bloodborne pathogens standard, following a baseline blood collection after an exposure incident at the dental office with the employee not giving consent to test for HIV, how long should the exposed employee's blood be preserved by the testing laboratory?

a. 40 days
b. 75 days
c. 90 days
d. 125 days

88. After an evaluation following an exposure incident at work, how long does the evaluating healthcare professional have to provide the exposed employee with a written opinion of the results?

a. 10 days
b. 15 days
c. 20 days
d. 25 days

89. The process of removing a bur before disassembling the handpiece from a dental unit is known as a:

a. work practice control.
b. engineering control.
c. safety control.
d. standard care control.

90. Which of the following is a requirement set in place by the OSHA Hazard Communications Standard?

a. SDS forms only come with products that are considered biologically hazardous in the dental office.

b. When a new SDS form is received by a dental office, it must be presented to all affected staff and reviewed before the product can be used.

c. SDS forms are optional safety documents that are provided by most manufacturing companies regarding the components of the specific product.

d. Employers must ensure that any SDS forms that come in with products are maintained and readily accessible to employees.

91. What does the acronym SDS stand for?
    a. Safety Data Sheet
    b. Subject to Data Specifications
    c. Safety During Shipment
    d. Safety Depends on Significance

92. Which of the following is a requirement that all dental employers develop, implement, and maintain in their dental offices?
    a. A product and chemical sharing plan and agreement
    b. A written hazard communications program
    c. A chemical ingredient breakdown list
    d. A carcinogenic product list

93. According to the hazard communication standard, when should employees have training on hazardous chemicals in the workplace?
    a. At initial employment
    b. Every month
    c. Every 3 months
    d. Every 6 months

94. How long must a dental employer keep the medical records of all employees?
    a. Only as long as the employee is actively employed at the clinic
    b. For 5 years after the employee is no longer employed at the clinic
    c. For 10 years plus the duration of employment at the clinic
    d. For 30 years plus the duration of employment at the clinic

95. According to the 2003 MMWR and NIOSH, which of the following is the advised protocol for a dental auxiliary to follow when assisting chairside with lasers in order to avoid the spread of infectious diseases and cross-contamination?
    a. Ensure there is a fan in the room for adequate air ventilation
    b. Double mask during laser procedures
    c. Use a N-95 respirator
    d. Follow standard precautions and use high filtration surgical masks and possibly face shields.

96. Which of the following safety measures should be followed when working with the curing light during procedures?
    a. There are no additional safety measures that must be taken when working with the curing light, the dental auxiliary must only follow standard precautions.
    b. The dental auxiliary should always wear utility gloves when handling the curing light to protect the skin from thermal rays.
    c. The dental auxiliary should avoid looking directly at the light emitted from the curing light.
    d. The dental auxiliary must ensure they are wearing eye protection and a facemask to protect themselves from the infectious odors emitted from the curing light.

97. What type(s) of personal protective equipment should be worn when the dental auxiliary is working with alginate impression material?
    a. Mask
    b. Mask and eyewear
    c. Mask, eyewear, and gloves
    d. No personal protective equipment is needed, as this is harmless when in powder form

98. Which of the following safety protocols should be followed in the event of a mercury spill in a dental office?
    a. The mercury should be absorbed by paper towels and thrown in the trash receptacle, and the area should be decontaminated with a high-level disinfectant.
    b. A mercury spill kit should be used to clean and decontaminate the area.
    c. The spill should be diluted with a basic cleaning compound and then the area should be wiped down with an intermediate-level disinfectant.
    d. Mercury specific sand should be placed over the mercury, swept up, and placed in the biohazardous waste container.

99. Which of the following is NOT included in the bloodborne pathogens exposure control plan that should be implemented at each dental office?
    a. Hepatitis B vaccination requirements
    b. Exposure determinations
    c. Hazardous waste disposal
    d. Exposure incident protocols

100. Which term is defined as: a specific eye, mouth, or other mucous membrane, non-intact skin, or parenteral contact with blood or other potentially infectious material that results from the performance of an employee's duties?
    a. Exposure incident
    b. Bloodborne pathogens standard
    c. Hazard contamination event
    d. Exposure control plan

Answers and Explanations

1. B: There are 4 stages that an individual who becomes infected with a disease typically moves through. The first stage is the incubation stage and is the time period from when the individual becomes infected to the time where he or she first starts to show symptoms. The prodromal stage is where the individual may start to show minor signs and symptoms indicating infection. The acute stage is where all of the symptoms are present and the person is the most contagious. If a patient presents for dental treatment during the acute stage, the appointment should be rescheduled due to the potential for disease transmission. The final stage is the convalescent stage, in which the individual starts to recover from the infection.

2. D: An asymptomatic carrier is an individual that is infected with a disease but who does not show any symptoms. This type of individual poses a danger to dental healthcare workers and the general public, due to the fact that he or she is infected with a contagious disease and has the capability to spread that infection. However, the person may not show any signs or symptoms of an infection and may not even know about the infection.

3. A: Standard precautions is a concept that is used in dentistry that states that all human body fluids and blood are to be treated as if they are infected with an infectious disease. The term 'universal precautions' was used in the past, but was expanded upon by adding in that secretions and excretions from humans should also fit into the category of body fluids that are capable of spreading infection. This also includes non-intact skin and mucous membranes. Dental healthcare workers should ensure that they are protecting themselves from these substances by utilizing the appropriate personal protective equipment.

4. B: Legionnaires' disease is a disease that is caused by an individual being exposed to the *Legionella pneumophila* bacteria. It can only be spread by aerosolization and aspiration of contaminated water. The disease was named after an outbreak that occurred in Philadelphia during an American Legion convention. Tetanus is a bacterial infection that is introduced into the body by a break in the skin or a wound. MRSA is also a bacterial infection that is caused by the *S. aureus* bacterium, which is commonly carried on the skin. This can get inside the body through a break in the skin and cause infection or may even cause infection on the outer surfaces of the skin. Hepatitis B is a blood-borne virus that attacks the liver, commonly introduced into the body by infected blood and/or body fluids.

5. A: When an individual is infected with syphilis, he has a bacterial infection that is caused by the *Treponema pallidum* spirochete bacteria. The bacteria enter the body through an open sore, through blood, or through body fluids. Once the infection starts, it can be divided into three stages. During the first stage, the infected individual may develop an ulcerating infectious sore called a chancre. The dental healthcare worker must prevent fluids from this lesion from contacting her skin or mucous membranes in order to prevent the spread of this infection. During the second stage, the infected individual may demonstrate mucous patches and measles-type rashes on the body. The third stage is typically fatal and does not show itself until 20 years after the initial infection, due to remaining dormant in the body for so many years.

6. A: There are a few different types of latex allergies, and with each type comes a different set of symptoms, some more severe than others. With a type 1 latex allergy or latex sensitivity, the affected patient or dental healthcare worker may start to show signs of an immune response

minutes or hours after the initial exposure. Common reactions include watery eyes, sneezing, and hives. There are more severe symptoms that have been demonstrated with a type 1 latex reaction including asthma, difficulty breathing, and in rare cases, there have been anaphylactic reactions and death. A dental healthcare worker must always know if she has a latex sensitivity or if her patients do in order to ensure that these types of situations do not happen.

7. A: According to the 2003 MMWR, since the 1980's, hepatitis B infections that were caused by exposure to blood or other potentially infectious materials at work via percutaneous exposure have decreased due to the rise in dental staff receiving vaccinations. Employers must offer the hepatitis B vaccine to all new employees at no charge; this vaccination is also discussed in the OSHA Blood-borne Pathogen Standard and is a main tool in preventing future hepatitis B infections. It is so important, that if a dental healthcare worker should decline this vaccination, they are required to sign a declination form stating they did not want to receive the vaccination and that they know the occupational risks of working with blood and body fluids.

8. D: The high volume evacuator is recommended for use if a patient is infected with a communicable disease due to the strong suction support that it provides and its ability to remove any airborne particles before they can be inhaled by the dental healthcare worker(s). Dry angles, small suction, and cotton roll holders are all useful tools during patient procedures and retraction techniques, but are not directly used to prevent the spread of disease transmission in dentistry.

9. D: Hepatitis C is a virus that can lead to chronic liver infections in 80% of the people that become infected. Chronic infections with hepatitis C may lead to cirrhosis of the liver and liver cancer with the potential for liver failure. This virus is spread by contact with contaminated blood and may be transmitted through childbirth from an infected mother, blood transfusions, organ transplants, and sexual intercourse. Hepatitis A is a virus that causes acute infections of the liver, rarely ever turning into chronic conditions and is caused by fecal contamination in the food and/or water supply. Shingles is a form of the herpes virus that leads to a very painful rash; and herpes type 1 is a virus that causes herpetic lesions, commonly known as cold sores on the oral mucosa and lips.

10. A: The hepatitis B vaccination is required for healthcare workers in the dental field. If a dental healthcare worker declines the vaccination, they must sign a declination form or a waiver, which will become a permanent part of their medical record kept by their employer. At this time, there are no booster doses recommended for the hepatitis B vaccine. This vaccine, which is composed of hepatitis B antigens, is given throughout a series of 3 injections: the initial dose; then 1 month later, the 2nd dose is administered; then 3 months later, the 3rd dose is administered. A titer test should be completed 1-2 months after the final dose to ensure the vaccination did cause the body to form antibodies to the hepatitis B virus.

11. C: The dental healthcare worker can only use liquid soap regardless of what type of procedure is being performed. Bar soap should never be used in a dental office as it can transmit infection by multiple people touching it. Hands should be washed with liquid soap both before donning gloves and after the removal of gloves due to small unapparent defects possibly being present in the gloves. Hands-free sinks also provide dental healthcare workers with the best option for avoiding cross-contamination, as workers no longer have to worry about touching contaminated faucets.

12. A: Alcohol-based hand rubs are a new category of hand hygiene products that are more effective at removing microbes from the hands than plain soap and some antimicrobial agents. In order to work effectively, the hands must not be visibly soiled or dirty, and the hand rub must have an

alcohol concentration of 60-95%. These are also very dose sensitive, so the dental healthcare worker must be sure to use the proper dose indicated by the manufacturer.

13. C: Petroleum-based products are not recommended for use in dentistry when used in conjunction with latex products, as the petroleum has the potential to break down the latex product making it less effective and increasing the chance for cross-contamination.

14. B: The CDC recommends that a dental healthcare worker avoid wearing artificial nails or nail extenders when providing patient care, especially to those patients who are at high risk. Natural nails should be kept at a length of less than ¼ inch, hand lotions and creams should be used to avoid dermatitis, and excessive drying of the hands may lead to cracked skin, which provides a portal of entry for microbes.

15. B: When working chairside, the dental healthcare worker should change his mask between every patient and more often if performing long procedures. This is due to patient fluids and saliva potentially splashing onto the dental mask and compromising its integrity. Standard dental masks filter out 95% of the particles they come into contact with, and in 1995, 2 other classes of dental masks were developed that filter out 99% and 99.97% of microbes they come into contact with. N-95 respirators are rarely used in the dental office as they require training and must be fit to the staff member.

16. A: Eyewear is a required piece of personal protective equipment that needs to be worn by all dental healthcare workers when performing chairside procedures, as well as laboratory and sterilization procedures. The dental healthcare worker may substitute a face shield in place of protective eyewear as long as that face shield is at least chin length and curved to offer the wearer side protection. The eyewear should be disinfected after every patient to avoid any cross-contamination.

17. C: In order to avoid cross-contamination, the correct order for the dental healthcare worker to put on personal protective equipment is protective clothing, eyewear, mask, and gloves. Gloves should always be put on last, as this will reduce the chances of the dental healthcare worker touching objects and then placing her gloves in the patient's mouth, which could lead to potential infections.

18. C: The dental healthcare worker should wear utility gloves when disinfecting treatment rooms and processing dental instruments. The purpose of wearing utility gloves is to provide additional protection against sharp objects and instruments. These gloves should never be worn during patient procedures, including exposing radiographs and performing laboratory duties. These gloves may also be disinfected and sterilized when needed.

19. C: Resident skin flora consists of bacteria that live on the skin and can never be completely removed. When washing hands, this type of bacteria can be reduced, but will never be completely gone, even with a stringent surgical scrub. These resident bacteria live in different layers of the skin, colonizing these layers. This type of bacteria does have the potential to cause disease, but are less likely to do so compared to other types of bacteria found on the hands.

20. B: The dental dam has a variety of benefits when used, both for the patient and for the dental healthcare worker. When considering the dental healthcare worker, the dental dam helps to protect him by reducing the amount of aerosols emitted into the air by the patient; this decreases the chance that the dental healthcare worker would breathe in an infectious substance and become ill.

This is also beneficial to the dental healthcare worker, as it discourages patient conversation and decreases the amount of time that may be needed to complete the procedure.

21. D: Single-use or disposable items are made to be used one time only. They are not to be cleaned, disinfected, or sterilized for a second use under any circumstances. Many products are made in disposable forms, which is very beneficial for hard-to-clean items. These items may increase the risk of cross-contamination when used, so a disposable alternative is a good choice. Single-use items are made of materials that cannot withstand the heat of a sterilizer and therefore should not be placed in such a device.

22. D: Pre-procedural mouth rinses have the purpose of reducing the number of microbes present in the mouth prior to a procedure being performed. This will then decrease the amount of microbes that have the potential to be released from the patient's mouth and into the air. According to the CDC, there is no substantial evidence indicating that pre-procedural mouth rinses reduce the prevalence of clinical infections, and therefore, they are not recommended for use at this time to prevent clinical infections among patients or dental healthcare workers.

23. A: When evaluating surgical smoke from electrosurgery procedures, tissue debris, viruses, and offensive odors have all been found to be present. If someone were to breathe in this surgical smoke, even with viruses being present, the rate of disease transmission is almost zero. There have been no cases of HIV or HBV transmission reported with this activity and there is no recommendation for testing from past exposures to this surgical smoke. The dental healthcare worker should follow standard precautions when performing these procedures.

24. D: When considering the use of single-dose vials of anesthetic in dentistry, the dental healthcare worker must understand that they are to never reuse any leftover materials, even if the needle on the syringe is changed. The vials pose a risk for contamination if they are repeatedly punctured and because of this, they should always be discarded after a single use.

25. B: When handling biopsy specimens, the items need to be in a container that is leak-proof, sturdy, and has a secure lid. This container must have a biohazard symbol on it as well during storage, transport, and disposal. The specimen should not be automatically kept in a refrigerator during storage unless indicated by the medical lab that is contracted with the dentist. Once a container has been used, it should be properly disposed of to avoid the potential of cross-contamination if that container were to be reused.

26. C: Prior to packaging a contaminated impression, the dental healthcare worker must first clean off the impression with soap and water to remove any blood or saliva that may be present. The impression then needs to be disinfected for the correct tuberculocidal time indicated by the manufacturer, and then rinsed. The impression is ready to be sent to the lab in a condition that will produce the least risk for cross-contamination between the dental office and the laboratory.

27. A: Touch surfaces are those that are directly touched and contaminated during treatment procedures. These surfaces include dental light handles, dental unit controls, chair switches, pens, containers of dental materials, and drawer handles. These differ from transfer surfaces in that transfer surfaces are not directly touched but are often touched by contaminated instruments. Transfer surfaces include instrument trays and handpiece holders.

28. B: One of the many advantages of using surface barriers in the dental office is that they protect hard-to-access areas that may not be easily cleaned and/or disinfected. If these areas can't be easily

accessed to be disinfected, the chances for cross-contamination increase. Barriers are less time consuming than pre-cleaning and disinfecting, and do not damage the equipment or surfaces as many of the disinfectants do after being used every day multiple times. Surface barriers do add waste to the environment though, as they can only be used once and then must be discarded.

29. C: The dental assistant should always be sure to change her gloves between patients, but it is also recommended that the dental assistant change her gloves when working on the same patient if the procedure is longer than one hour. If the dental assistant has to leave the room during a procedure, she should always remove her gloves and wash her hands prior to exiting the treatment room, as it is not acceptable to walk around with contaminated gloves. Under no circumstances should the dental assistant ever wash her gloves. If a contaminated object has touched the gloves, the dental assistant needs to remove the gloves, wash her hands, and place on a new pair of gloves prior to returning to patient care.

30. C: When considering the cleaning and disinfection of housekeeping surfaces, is it important to know that these are the areas in the dental office that pose little risk in the transmission of disease. These areas need to only be cleaned with a hospital-grade disinfectant or a low-level disinfectant. Walls and drapery items do not need to be cleaned unless they are visibly contaminated. If mops and cloths are used to disinfect any areas, they should immediately be cleaned and allowed to dry prior to use to prevent any cross-contamination between areas.

31. B: Regulated biohazardous waste is the type of waste that is produced in the dental office and must be disposed of in a special manner due to the ability of this type of waste to spread infection. Examples of regulated biohazardous waste include blood-soaked items, items with dried blood that is flaking off, items saturated with other body fluids, and extracted teeth.

32. C: Biohazardous waste items including extracted teeth, items saturated with blood and body fluids, and items caked with dried blood must be disposed of in a regulated biohazardous waste container. This container must be labeled with a biohazardous waste sticker, and is meant for non-sharp items. When placing items in this container, the dental healthcare worker must ensure the items do not contaminate the outside of the container.

33. A: A sharps container should never be filled past capacity; the dental healthcare worker needs to remove the sharps container from use prior to the items filling the entire container. If this is allowed to happen, the chances of the dental healthcare worker obtaining a percutaneous injury increase. When the sharps container is nearing full capacity, the container should be closed and removed from the operatory for final disposal.

34. C: When placing biohazardous waste into a biohazard bag and the bag becomes contaminated, the dental healthcare worker should place the entire contaminated bag into a second biohazardous bag and seal both bags. If the bags were to be wiped down, or emptied into a new bag, the chances of cross-contamination increase and put the dental healthcare worker at greater risk for an occupational exposure. Not everyone who comes into contact with regulated waste bags and containers wear personal protective equipment, so a contaminated bag cannot be ignored, it must be handled properly.

35. D: Items that should be placed into a sharps container include used needles, burs, orthodontic bands and wires, and other sharp items. These containers are puncture resistant, leakage proof, and are intended to provide a safe, sturdy storage location for these sharp items and will keep these

items out of the regular trash where they are more likely to cause an occupational exposure or end up in landfills.

36. D: The dental healthcare worker should avoid storing instruments in areas where they can get wet, including under sinks. If the instrument pouches or paper become wet, wicking occurs, where microbes are actually able to pass through the wrapping and possibly contaminate the sterile instruments. It is helpful to label instruments with the date that they were sterilized; a permanent marker works best for this as it is easily visible, and it is good practice to store sterilized instruments in closed or covered cabinets, as these keep microbes that may be in the air away from the instruments. Both paper with autoclave tape and paper/plastic combinations are good choices to consider when selecting a packaging for instruments, as both of these keep instruments sterile after they have been in a sterilization machine.

37. C: Spent or used fixer is a type of hazardous waste because it has silver particles in it due to the reaction that occurs with the fixer and the emulsions found on dental radiographic films. A dental office must work with a hazardous waste disposal company and ensure that this product is being picked up and disposed of properly.

38. B: Cross-contamination is also known as indirect contact or indirect disease transmission. This occurs when a patient or dental healthcare worker is exposed to a contaminated instrument or any other contaminated item that was improperly processed and/or sterilized. It is important that the dental healthcare worker know the proper disinfection and sterilization protocols to follow in the dental setting to prevent indirect disease transmission from occurring.

39. D: The term parenteral means through the skin, so parenteral disease transmission occurs through a break in the skin. This may occur in the dental office when a person sticks himself with a contaminated needle, cuts himself with orthodontic arch wire, or any other way that the skin is punctured or cut. The dental healthcare worker must be mindful of the procedures he is performing and must be aware of the proper ways to handle these sharp items to avoid this situation.

40. C: Tuberculosis is a bacterial infection that is transferred through the air. When an infected individual coughs, sings, or speaks, this bacterium has the potential to enter the air. Once airborne, it may stay present in the air for hours, presenting the opportunity for other individuals to re-breathe the bacteria and become infected with tuberculosis.

41. B: Semi-critical instruments are those items that enter a patient's oral cavity but do not penetrate bone. These items should be sterilized by heat when possible, but when this is not an option, these items should be processed using a high-level disinfectant because this high-level disinfectant is capable of sterilization. Critical items penetrate bony tissue and must be sterilized by heat, and non-critical items do not come into contact with the oral cavity and therefore can be decontaminated using an intermediate or low-level disinfectant.

42. D: Sterilization can be described as the destruction of all living microorganisms. An item is either sterile or it is not, there is no in-between. When an item is disinfected, most forms of microorganisms are destroyed but the stronger microbes, including spores, may still be living on the item or surface. Critical level and semi-critical level instruments must be sterilized prior to being reused to avoid cross-contamination.

43. B: High-level disinfectants are those disinfectants that are capable of sterilization when the submersion time is greatly increased. Glutaraldehyde and chlorine dioxide are examples of

chemicals that can be used as methods of sterilization when items are submerged in these solutions for 6-10 hours, depending on the manufacturer's instructions. These items can also be used as disinfectants when needed.

44. B: When a disinfectant claims to have a tuberculocidal claim of 3 minutes, this means that the disinfectant is capable of killing the tuberculosis bacteria and all less-resistant forms of microbes in 3 minutes. When used, these products must remain on the surface for a minimum of three minutes, and the surface must remain wet for this amount of time as well, otherwise the disinfectant may not be effective in killing the tuberculosis bacteria.

45. D: When a noncritical item comes into contact with blood or body fluids, an intermediate or low-level disinfectant should be used to decontaminate the item prior to its next use. Many noncritical items are unable to withstand heat sterilization and will become damaged if placed in a sterilization machine. Many of these items are unable to withstand being submerged in a high-level disinfectant as well; therefore, they should be wiped down with an intermediate-level disinfectant, and allowed to remain wet for the correct tuberculocidal time prior to use on another patient.

46. D: A dental handpiece is an example of a semi-critical level instrument. The description of this category of instruments is that they come into contact with the mucosa in the oral cavity, but they do not penetrate bone. The bur that is placed in the dental handpiece would be considered a critical level instrument, but the handpiece itself is an example of a semi-critical level instrument.

47. D: The correct method of decontamination of a handpiece is that it should be wiped off with an intermediate-level disinfectant using disposable gauze and then bagged and placed in the sterilization machine used in the dental office. It is important that handpieces never be submerged in any solution, including that of the ultrasonic machine. This is because the liquid would damage the delicate parts of the motor in the handpiece.

48. A: A stethoscope is an example of a noncritical level instrument. This level of instrument can be described as one that comes into contact with intact skin and includes other items such as blood pressure cuffs and pulse oximeters. These items can be processed using an intermediate to low-level disinfectant.

49. C: The main purpose of the holding solution used in a dental sterilization area is to prevent the organic debris, the bioburden, from drying onto the instruments. If this material does dry onto the instruments, it can interfere with the sterilization process by creating a shelter for the microbes to hide in and preventing the sterilization machine from producing steam, heat, or a chemical vapor that can reach these microbes, rendering the item unsterile and leading to cross-contamination during patient care.

50. D: Ethylene oxide is a gas that is capable of sterilization using low temperatures, and is commonly used in large hospital settings. This method of sterilization works well for items that would melt in heat sterilization machines, but due to the long time requirement that is needed for this method, it is rarely found in a smaller dental practice setting. The ethylene oxide gas can take 4-12 hours to sterilize and then the instruments must be allowed to go through an aeration cycle to avoid burning patient tissue; this time period can range from 4-12 hours.

51. D: The ultrasonic machine is the most desirable form of pre-cleaning dental instruments in the dental office. This is because this is a hands-free way to ensure that the bioburden and any other debris are removed from the dental instruments prior to sterilization in a safe way. These cleaners

reduce the risk of percutaneous exposures to the hands during instrument processing because the dental healthcare worker simply places the contaminated instruments into the ultrasonic machine and starts the machine. When it has run its full cycle, the dental healthcare worker can pull out the basket containing the instruments and place them on the counter after they have been rinsed, removing the occupational risk for an injury by a dental instrument.

52. B: The foil test is an important test that must be completed on the ultrasonic machines to ensure that they are working properly and removing the bioburden from the instruments. It is a simple test where the dental healthcare worker places a piece of foil into the machine and holds part of it submerged for 20 seconds. The foil can then be removed and examined. If the ultrasonic machine is working properly, there should be uniform pitting, pebbling, and indentations across the part of the foil that was submerged in the machine.

53. C: The flash cycle, which is available on most models of sterilization machines, is intended for use when items in the cycle are to be used immediately after the cycle has been run. These cycles are shorter than the regular cycles because the instruments do not require packaging during the flash cycle. If an item is not used immediately after this cycle and is stored or put away for later use, there is the risk that the item will become contaminated because there is no packaging to prevent exposure to microbes in the environment.

54. A: Biological monitoring is the best way to ensure that a sterilization unit is functioning as it should in order to remove all microbes from the instruments placed into the machine. Biological monitoring involves the use of spore strips, which commonly contain the bacteria *Bacillus stearothermophilus* for steam units and *Bacillus subtilis* for dry heat units. These spore strips are placed inside the units along with a normal load of contaminated instruments and the machine is run as it normally would be. The spore strip is then sent out to a lab for processing or the dental office may use spore vials and process these vials in house. These strips or vials are tested to ensure that the bacteria contained on them has been destroyed by the sterilization machine.

55. D: Biological indicators are also referred to as spore tests. This is because these items contain spores, which are very resistant forms of microbes, and if these spores can be destroyed by the tested method of sterilization, then all weaker forms of microbes that may be present on the instruments will be destroyed as well.

56. A: Biofilms can be defined as the colonization of bacteria, fungi, and protozoa microbes that are found to live inside a protective slime layer, which is commonly found inside dental unit water lines. Biofilms do form in all water environments, but due to how dental unit water lines deliver water directly into a patient's mouth, the level of bacteria in these devices must be monitored and regulated to prevent unnecessary complications in dental patients.

57. C: The Environmental Protection Agency has set the maximum level of colony-forming units that can be found in dental treatment water at 500 CFU/mL. It is desired that manufacturing companies create devices that keep these levels below 300 CFU/mL, but the maximum amount allowed is set at 500 CFU/mL.

58. B: After each patient is seen in the dental office, the dental auxiliary should run any dental device that was used in the mouth and connected to a water system for a minimum of 20-30 seconds in order to flush out any patient material or bioburden that may have entered the dental waterline tubing. They should not be run with bleach, as this has not been demonstrated as an

effective way to clean the tubing, and simply flushing the lines at the beginning of the day does not affect the biofilm; this is not a reliable method to clean the dental water line tubing.

59. D: It is very important that when performing surgical procedures, the dental team uses sterile water if needed during the procedures. In order to prevent infection, the dental team also must ensure that this sterile water is reaching the surgical site in a sterile manner and is not being contaminated by bioburden, biofilms, or other microbial sources.

60. A: In the event that a city or community in which a dental office is located issues a boil-water advisory, it is important that the dental team know the proper protocol to follow to avoid putting their patients at risk for infections due to contaminated water. If this were to occur, the dental office should avoid using water from the public water supply for all patient procedures, both surgical and basic types. The dental team must avoid using water from faucets for handwashing as well, as this may contaminate their hands; bottled water can be used during these events for rinsing.

61. A: It is important for the dental auxiliary to ensure they are taking the proper steps to prevent the spread of disease to dental laboratory workers who come into contact with patient impressions and registrations. The dental auxiliary must be sure to disinfect all impressions with an intermediate-level disinfectant prior to sending them to the dental laboratory. While this will not remove all microbes from the impression, it will remove many microbes that could pose a risk to the dental lab workers. If metal trays are used, they must be sterilized prior to reuse. It is important that the dental office and laboratory have an understanding of who is responsible for the final disinfection of the patient items; one cannot always assume that the other will disinfect the final product before it is placed on the patient.

62. C: There are many different types of disinfectant choices to consider when deciding how to disinfect impression materials. The best choices for alginate impressions are iodophors and dilute sodium hypochlorite solution. There are many products available that contain these chemicals, so the dental office can decide as a team which product works best for their office.

63. C: Prior to performing an oral surgical procedure, the dental auxiliary must ensure they are decontaminating their hands properly in order to prevent the spread of infection. The use of antimicrobial soap alone and rinsing with tap water is an acceptable practice and can be used prior to both basic and surgical procedures. The dental auxiliary can also use plain soap and water followed by an alcohol-based hand scrub.

64. C: The best and most effective way for a dental auxiliary to prevent cross-contamination from occurring during the use of digital radiographic sensors is to place the sensor(s) in barriers during use, and afterwards, wipe down the sensor(s) with an intermediate-level disinfectant. These sensors are unable to be sterilized, as the heat, steam, and/or chemicals will damage the delicate parts, nor can these items be submerged in any type of liquid.

65. A: When using any type of film positioning device, it should be sterilized by heat if it is able to withstand the high temperatures by using an autoclave or chemiclave as both use high temperatures to sterilize. These items are semi-critical level instruments so they do need to be sterilized, but in the event that they are not able to withstand high temperatures, many types may be submerged in a high-level disinfectant that is capable of sterilization.

66. C: The most effective way to prevent cross-contamination from occurring when using radiographic films on patients is to wrap each individual film in a barrier before it goes into the

mouth and then remove each film from the barrier after it has been removed from the mouth. This prevents the patient's tissue and saliva from ever coming into contact with the film and will allow the dental auxiliary to process the film with minimal contamination to the processing units.

67. D: When decontaminating an area on the floor in a treatment room after a blood spill, the dental auxiliary must use a disinfectant that has a tuberculocidal time. Therefore, intermediate or high-level disinfectants must be used, as low-level disinfectants are not capable of killing tuberculosis. These intermediate-level disinfectants need to be used on clinical contact surfaces with or without visible blood.

68. D: When considering which disinfectants to use in a dental office, the dental team must know that in order to be used in dentistry, whichever disinfectant they select must have an Environmental Protection Agency (EPA) registration number. Without this number, regardless of the claims of the product, it cannot be used in the dental office. Different disinfectants will have different tuberculocidal kill times so there is not a specific number that must be met, nor do the disinfectants need to be listed on the American Dental Association's website.

69. B: There are a variety of reasons as to why a sterilization unit would fail to sterilize the instruments that are found inside, but the main reason for sterilization failure is error on the operator's behalf. The machine may have been loaded too full, the operator may have used incorrect packaging, the incorrect cycle was selected, or excessive packaging may have been used. The dental auxiliary must ensure they are following proper procedures when using the sterilization units to prevent these situations from occurring.

70. B: Once a city or municipality has lifted a boil-water advisory, the dental office must follow certain steps prior to using city water from the faucets. Specific action must be completed unless otherwise directed by public officials. The dental office must flush the dental unit water lines for 1-5 minutes prior to using any tap water during patient procedures and washing hands. There is no need to remove any dental hoses from the operatory, as these hoses are not able to withstand the heat that is used when sterilization occurs in the autoclave, nor does this tubing need to be soaked in any type of disinfectant.

71. A: Engineering controls are pieces of equipment or devices that need to be used in dental offices in order to prevent exposure to items that may be contaminated with bloodborne pathogens. These controls make procedures safer for dental team members and decrease the chances that a dental team worker sustains any type of percutaneous injury. Examples include handwashing stations, sharps containers, eye washing stations, and needle recapping devices.

72. A: The bloodborne pathogens standard is set in place to help protect all employees who are exposed to blood or other potentially infectious materials. This standard has many areas of coverage that relate to different fields in which workers may come into contact with blood, including nursing, dentistry, and mortuary science. All individuals in these fields are expected to abide by and follow the guidelines in this standard.

73. B: The exposure control plan is a plan that needs to be developed and implemented in each dental office and has the intent of eliminating or minimizing employee exposure to blood or other potentially infectious materials. This needs to be accessible by all employees and does not need to be filed with OSHA, but must be available if requested during an audit.

74. C: Each dental office must ensure that their exposure control plan is reviewed and updated annually. It should also be reviewed and updated if there are new or modified tasks and procedures, which may affect occupational exposures at work or if there are new positions that have been created.

75. B: The occupational exposure determination is part of the bloodborne pathogens standard and is an element of the exposure control plan in which the employer must identify workers who have an occupational risk of coming into contact with blood or other potentially infectious materials. The office must identify job classifications in which all of the employees have occupational exposure (doctor) and also job classifications in which some of the employees have occupational exposure (hospital laundry worker).

76. D: According to the bloodborne pathogens standard, employers shall provide handwashing stations that are readily accessible to employees. Employers can't simply decide not to install handwashing facilities, as these are a vital engineering control and are a main factor in the prevention of disease transmission at the dental office. There may be a time where the dental auxiliary is not able to use the handwashing station, and should then have the ability to use antiseptic hand cleaners or towelettes, but hands should then be washed with soap and water as soon as feasible.

77. D: Upon initial employment at a dental office, the employer must offer the new employee the hepatitis B vaccination at no cost to the employee within 10 days. If the employee initially declines the series, they may change their mind at a later date with the employer still being responsible for the cost of the series. If an employee declines to receive the vaccination, they must sign a declination form, which will become part of their permanent medical record; there is no required counseling if this were to occur.

78. B: The optimal time for an employee to receive a titer test and determine if there was antibody development as a result of the hepatitis B vaccine is 1-2 months after the final dose of the series has been administered. This will determine if the employee is protected or if they must be revaccinated and retested.

79. B: If an employee receives 2 sets of the hepatitis B vaccination series and does not respond with antibody production after these sets, they are known as a non-responder and are considered to be susceptible to acquiring a hepatitis B infection. These individuals should be counseled to ensure that they are aware of their status and that they follow proper protocol in the event where they are involved in an exposure at work. It is not advised that they receive the series a 3rd time, and they need not be removed from their current position as long as they are aware of the risks they face due to their status as a non-responder.

80. A: The employer is responsible for providing personal protective equipment to the employees at no cost. This includes gloves, masks, eye protection, and smocks, gowns, or scrubs. The employer is not able to charge the employee if they experience an allergic reaction to certain protective devices; instead, the employer must provide an alternative form of protection to the employee. If a piece of personal protective equipment is damaged due to incorrect cleaning procedures, the employee should be counseled on how to use that item properly, but is not responsible for replacing the item.

81. A: In the event that there is broken glass in any location within a dental clinic, the dental auxiliary or staff members involved should not pick up the glass directly with their hands. A brush and dustpan, tongs, or forceps should be used to clean up the glass and then place it directly into a

sharps container to prevent any other employees from coming into contact with the glass and possibly puncturing their skin.

82. B: An item is considered infectious regulated waste if it is caked with blood that can be released from the item if the item is compressed and also if there is dried blood that is flaking off of the item. If an item has a small amount of blood on it, such as a Band-Aid or a patient napkin, this type of waste can be deposited into a regular trash receptacle. If there is infectious waste generated by a dental office, this type of waste must be removed by a waste disposal company who is licensed to handle the specific type of waste, and records must be kept to demonstrate this disposal.

83. D: According to the bloodborne pathogens standard, contaminated work surfaces should be cleaned or decontaminated after completion of a procedure, immediately or as soon as possible after there has been a spill of blood or any other type of potentially infectious material, or at the end of a work shift if the area in question has been contaminated since the last cleaning. A procedure does not need to be stopped if an area becomes contaminated with saliva as this can wait until the procedure is over.

84. C: Infectious waste is a type of regulated waste that is produced in dentistry and includes items such as extracted teeth and non-intact patient tissues. This type of waste should always be placed in containers that are closable, and that are constructed to contain all contents during handling, storage, transport, and shipping. General and contaminated waste can be placed in a regular trash receptacle when produced in dentistry and includes items such as saliva-soaked gauze and contaminated patient napkins. Specialized waste is not a recognized type of waste produced in the dental field.

85. A: When handling the contaminated laundry that is generated by a dental office, the team member or dental auxiliary must wear protective gloves and other appropriate personal protective equipment when necessary to protect themselves against blood or other potentially infectious material. If the laundry is wet, it must be placed and transported in bags or containers that prevent soak-through from occurring. If it is laundered on site, any team member is capable of assisting in washing items, it is not solely the responsibility of the dentist.

86. D: According to the bloodborne pathogens standard, following a report of an exposure incident occurring in a dental clinic, the employer is required to provide a confidential medical evaluation and follow-up to the exposed employee, performed by a qualified physician. This includes blood testing on the exposed individual to determine if they have been infected with hepatitis B or HIV. Documentation must be taken regarding the route of exposure and the circumstances under which the exposure incident occurred.

87. C: After a baseline blood collection is taken, if the employee does not give consent to test his blood for HIV, the sample should be preserved for at least 90 days. If the employee changes his mind and decides to have the baseline sample tested, the blood will be available.

88. B: Following an exposure incident at the dental office, the exposed employee will be sent to a physician for post-exposure follow-up and testing. The employer must obtain and provide those results to the affected employee within 15 days of the completion of the evaluation. This is set in place to ensure that results are given within a timely manner and to aid in the event that additional steps are required due to an acquired infection from an occupational exposure at work.

89. A: The process of removing a bur before disassembling the handpiece from a dental unit is known as a work practice control. This type of procedure is set in place to protect dental workers. Other examples include restricting the use of fingers during tissue or cheek retraction and using a mouth mirror or other instrument instead, and minimizing the uncontrolled movement of scalers or laboratory knives during use. If followed, work practice controls will help to reduce the occupational exposure to sharp items experienced by dental team members.

90. D: According to the hazard communications standard, employers must ensure that any SDS forms that come in with products are maintained and readily accessible to employees. This is important in the event that there was a chemical spill or exposure, in that these forms could be easily accessed to aid in guiding clean-up or decontamination procedures. SDS forms are required for each product and as long as the product is in the office, the SDS form must be kept on hand, either electronically or physically. When new SDS forms arrive, they can be uploaded or filed and reviewed as needed by employees; there is no need to alert all employees of a new form.

91. A: The acronym SDS (formerly MSDS) stands for Safety Data Sheet. The SDS is a document that is sent along with all hazardous products that are used in a dental office setting. The SDS form has a wide range of information on it that may be beneficial in the event of a product or chemical spill or if an employee comes into physical contact with a hazardous chemical. There are decontamination and clean-up procedures listed on these forms, along with the chemical nature of the product. The dental team member can also find routes of entry and affected organs on these forms.

92. B: According to the hazard communications standard, each dental office must develop, implement, and maintain a written hazard communications program, which describes how training needs will be met, how SDS forms are to be handled and accessed, and a list of hazardous products. There is no need or requirement to have a specific list of carcinogenic products, a chemical sharing plan, or a chemical ingredient breakdown list.

93. A: The hazard communications standard requires that employers provide employees with information and training on hazardous products in their work area at the time of initial employment and when a new hazard is present that the employee has not been trained on in the past. This will ensure the employee is aware of the hazards in the workplace and also that they know the location of the written hazard communications program and the hazardous chemical list.

94. D: According to the bloodborne pathogens standard, a dental employer must keep all employees medical records for at least the duration of employment plus 30 years. This is a mandated requirement that all dental employers must follow. It is important that the employing dentist have all the pertinent medical records in this file including vaccination records and any exposure incident forms.

95. D: According to the 2003 MMWR, when working with lasers, there is the potential for the thermal description of tissues to create a smoke byproduct that has the capability of containing particles, gases, tissue debris, viruses, and offensive odors. NIOSH recommends that those who are exposed to this smoke follow standard precautions and use high-filtration surgical masks and possibly full-face shields to protect themselves.

96. C: When working with a curing light during any type of procedure, the dental auxiliary must always remember to never look directly at the light emitted from the curing light. This is because this light has the potential to damage the retina of the eyes. The dental auxiliary does not need to

wear any additional personal protective equipment when using this device, as it does not emit any offensive odors that require extra protection.

97. C: When working with alginate material, the dental auxiliary must wear a mask, eyewear, and gloves to protect themselves from the fine powders that may be released as they are preparing the alginate material for use. It is good practice to always wear gloves when working with dental products to prevent these products from being absorbed into the skin, and also to wear eyewear to prevent anything from splashing into the eyes.

98. B: In the event of a mercury spill in a dental office, the dental auxiliary should use the mercury spill kit, which every dental office should have on hand to clean and decontaminate the area. This spill kit should include items that are specific to cleaning this hazardous chemical, including mercury-absorbing powder, mercury-absorbing sponges, and a disposal bag for the waste. The dental auxiliary must always wear eye protection, a mask, and utility gloves when cleaning a mercury spill.

99. C: A bloodborne pathogens exposure control plan should include exposure determinations, methods of compliance with the plan, hepatitis B vaccination records and any other vaccination records, engineering controls, and work practice controls. Hazardous waste disposal is not part of the bloodborne pathogens standard and therefore is not included in this plan. This type of waste disposal includes used and outdated chemicals and is discussed and covered under the hazard communications standard, as it does not involve infectious waste disposal.

100. A: An exposure incident can be defined as a specific eye, mouth, or other mucous membrane, non-intact skin, or parenteral contact with blood or other potentially infectious material that results from the performance of an employee's duties. This incident would then be documented and evaluated using the exposure control plan set in place at the location of the event. This is part of the bloodborne pathogens standard, which all dental offices must follow in order to be in compliance with OSHA.